The 8 Laws of Chiropractic Success

Powerful Insights Into Personal and Professional Transformation

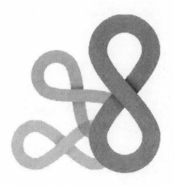

David K. Scheiner, D.C.

With A Foreword by Wayne Dyer
Author of Your Erroneous Zones

NATURALLY WELL PUBLICATIONS, LLC
Phoenix, Arizona

The 8 Laws of Chiropractic Success

Powerful Insights Into
Personal and Professional Transformation
by Dr. David K. Scheiner

Published by:
Naturally Well Publications, LLC
Phoenix, AZ

ISBN: 978-1-7323632-4-3

First Printing: June 2018

Printed in the United States of America

Additional copies of this book may be ordered at:
www.DavidScheiner.com/Books

Design by Marty Marsh
www.SupportedSelfPublishing.com

All photographs are used with the permission
of the respective copyright holders.

Praise for
The 8 Laws of Chiropractic

"You hold in your hands a 'must read' chiropractic success manual collected from the best and brightest minds in the profession. Dr. David K. Scheiner's **The 8 Laws of Chiropractic Success** probes and dissects the consciousness that drives them. This brilliant anthology is jam-packed with the clues needed to realize and experience this awesome thing we call "success in chiropractic!" Invest your time reading it — you're worth it." — Billy DeMoss, D.C., founder of Cal Jam, Dead Chiropractic Society, and DeMoss Chiropractic

"The 8 Laws probe the very heart of what's happening with chiropractors and students today! A 'must read' book for every D.C. and student who cares about their current and future success in Life and chiropractic practice." — Steve Judson, D.C., owner of Judson Family Chiropractic and author of **Atlas Adjusted** and **Wake Up Human**s

"Dr. David K. Scheiner managed to get some of the top chiropractic leaders to talk candidly about the most important success principles chiropractors and students must implement today." — Paul Reed, D.C., founder of Chiro-Fest and Bridge Chiropractic

"A wonderful collection of intriguing chiropractic figures brought together for one book. Their contributions will spark growth, inspiration, and success." — Tim Young, D.C., president of Focus OKC and Focus Foundations

"Inspiring stories, enlightening principles, and time-tested actions that will help chiropractors serve even more millions of patients." — John F. Demartini, D.C., founder of the Demartini Institute and the bestselling author of "Count Your Blessings"

"An Absolutely compelling book! It's like sitting in a room full of chiropractic legends and learning what it takes to become great in life and chiropractic practice. Amazing stuff." — Gilles LaMarche, D.C., VP of Professional Relations at Life University

"Kudos to David Scheiner for bringing together, in one place, the insights of some of chiropractic's greatest minds. By reading this book and implementing the wisdom of **The 8 Laws of Chiropractic Success**, you will realize massive achievement."— Daniel and Richelle Knowles, D.C.'s, founders of Mile High Chiro

"A perfect recipe for success, blending fascinating personal wisdom with perceptive expert opinions." — Ross McDonald and Rebecca Vickery, D.C.'s, founders of The Edinburgh Lectures

"A printed Mastermind Meeting! Chock full of concepts and visions—sure to inspire you with the wisdom to build a successful life of significance." — D.D. Humber, D.C., 1956 graduate of Palmer College and former host of Dynamic Essentials Seminars for over 50 years

"Reading these chiropractors' experiences connects us to the roots of eternal success, rekindles our passion, and inspires our vision for future achievement in chiropractic."— Brad Glowaki, D.C., founder of Glowaki Chiropractic and New Patient Maven

"Dr. Scheiner's book is an incredible compilation of insights and stories from chiropractic leaders and legends. I am amazed by the wisdom and passion that leaps out from every page. This should be required reading for every chiropractor and every chiropractic student!" — Cathy Wendland-Colby, D.C., founder and CEO of the Women Speakers Club and Colby Family Chiropractic

"This book realizes the famous time-tested principles of chiropractic success passed down from generation to generation from those who've led the great chiropractic life." — Frederick A. Schofield, D.C., founder of Schofield Chiropractic Training

"A great balance of profound success principles and reflective personal insights." — Guy Riekeman, D.C., Chancellor, Life University

"A current viewpoint from leaders who've influenced the development of chiropractic and will inspire current and future chiropractors to grow both personally and professionally." — Jessica Harden, D.C., founder of Providence Chiropractic and FLIGHT

"By reading and implementing the fascinating lessons in this book, you are making a great investment in your personal life, professional success, and in the future healing of humanity." — Donny Epstein, D.C., founder of Network Spinal Analysis, Reorganizational Healing, and EpiEnergetics

"This is a great book that intertwines chiropractic success principles and rich chiropractic personalities into a marvelous readable style. It is a must read for every chiropractor, student, or retired D.C." — Amanda & Jeremy Hess, D.C.'s, founders of AMPED and Discover Chiropractic

"A brilliant gathering of some of the greatest minds in the chiropractic profession – providing insights into what it takes to see more people and remove more subluxations." — Jim Dubel, D.C., founder of New Beginnings Chiropractic Philosophy Weekend

"Unlike my first book Chiropractic Revealed, **The 8 Laws of Chiropractic Success** exposes the arrows pointing directly at the target of success in both chiropractic and Life." — David K. Scheiner, D.C., author of **Chiropractic Revealed** and founder of **The 5 FLAGS of Transformation**

Contents

Acknowledgements 6

Dedication 8

About the Author: *David K. Scheiner, D.C.* 9

Foreword *by Wayne Dyer* 11

Introduction 21

THE LAWS

    Law One – Mindset 27

    Law Two – Vision 59

    Law Three – Intention 87

    Law Four – Service 115

    Law Five – Rejection 139

    Law Six – Love 167

    Law Seven – Giving 191

    Law Eight – Action 213

About the Contributors 237

Conclusion 253

Acknowledgements

This is my second book for the chiropractic profession and I've chosen to use the same graphic and design wizard again. Marty Marsh is a creative genius who I owe so much. Thank you Marty. I must also thank my superstar editor, Barbara Bigham, who edited a portion of this book and then passed on too soon for so many of us. You live on in this book Barbara and I thank you.

Hopefully, you too have people in your life that provide unconditional support with every idea you bring to them (and I have many). That's what I have with my wife of over twenty years. Thank you Laura for always listening, for providing unwavering support and encouragement, and for being an incredible mother. I also give so much thanks to my three beautiful girls (now all grown up) Megan, Kira, and Summer for always sticking by my side and for being beacons of light and hope for the future of humanity.

This book, as you will see, is comprised of contributions from many of the leaders within the chiropractic profession and I'd like to thank each one of them for taking the time out of their already packed schedules to participate and play here. Your words within this volume will assist many chiropractors, their offices, and chiropractic students to realize a great, great life.

This book would not have come to life if it were not for D.D. and B.J. Palmer, D.C.'s, who discovered and developed the Chiropractic profession respectively. It would not have come to life if it were not for Sid E Williams, D.C., who pierced my soul and brought me to Life Chiropractic College in 1992. This book would not have come to life if not for the late Reggie Gold and

James Sigafoose, D.C.'s, mentors who taught me so much and who also devoted their entire existence to chiropractic. And this book certainly would not have come to life if not for the communication brilliance of Guy Riekeman, Arno Burnier, and Donny Epstein, D.C.'s., who instilled their principles of work ethic and authenticity in me. All the names in this paragraph imprinted their chiropractic genius within me and for that I remain eternally grateful. So, thank you!

▦

In Loving Memory of
My Father-In-Law

Edward W. Mihalek, Ph.D

(November 1, 1941 – May 2, 2018)

▦

Dedication

This book is dedicated to all the souls who are wise enough to lay on a chiropractic table and to those who have enough courage, grit, and fortitude to lay their hands on them.

About The Author

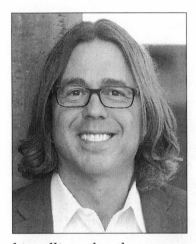

Originally from Queens, N.Y., Dr. David Scheiner grew up in Roslyn, Long Island. It was a unique and special place. He was spiritual from the outset; constantly challenging the status-quo, while marveling at the wonders of the universe and how he fit into its schematics.

Knowing that his purpose from an early age was to help people at a high-level, chiropractic became his calling when he sent away for information from Life Chiropractic College in 1992. It was when he read Dr. Sid Williams' presidents message in the college handbook, that he had an awakening. The Universe immediately called him to action to become a chiropractor. He fell in love with Dr. Sid's Native American and philosophical messages and became a 1996 graduate of Life Chiropractic College (now Life University) in Marietta, GA.

He remained in Atlanta for twenty-two years and opened four highly-successful chiropractic clinics with his wife Laura, a highly sought-after pediatric and pregnancy chiropractor. During this period, David developed and implemented wellness programs for Fortune 500 companies in Atlanta, GA. The Home Depot, GE, IBM, Colgate Palmolive, Delta Airlines, and The Weather Channel are a few he worked with and positively impacted.

In 2012, David went to work with Life Chiropractic College West in Hayward, CA and as Director of Recruitment helped take new student enrollment to healthy new heights. David remains committed to introducing prospective students to chiropractic colleges even though he is no longer with Life Chiropractic College West.

He is a teacher of meditation, student of the esoteric and mystical arts, sought after lecturer, and author of two books — **Chiropractic Revealed**, an interview compilation including some of the most well-known chiropractors to ever grace the profession and — this volume, **The 8 Laws of Chiropractic Success**. He is currently working on his newest book The 5 FLAGS of Transformation along with its accompanying workbook and growthshops. The 5 FLAGS of Transformation movement is slated for world-wide release in late 2019.

David and his wife Laura currently reside in Phoenix, Arizona and have three beautiful daughters; Megan, Kira, and Summer and two incredible dogs, Charlie and Henri.

Learn more about David at: www.davidscheiner.com

Foreword

Wayne Dyer, Ph.D.

Thank you, David for giving me the opportunity to contribute to chiropractors, chiropractic students, and the chiropractic profession. The chiropractic profession holds many wonderful attributes within its grasp and it is only when it gets out of its own way that those attributes may be unleashed; unveiling it's great promises for all of humanity to experience.

Where you've caught me right now is over on Marko Island in South West Florida, where I'm writing this new book which has a lot to do with many of the topics you've slated for this new book, "The 8 Laws of Chiropractic Success." I'm so happy to contribute so let's get right to it shall we?

Mindset

Virtually, anything that you put your mind to I believe you have the power to create. I've been practicing that all of my life. This new book I'm writing right now is really about the idea of being able to put your attention on what it is that you want to manifest and practicing these certain principles, which I've sort of been doing unconsciously since I was a little boy. When you do practice these principles, you can really attract to yourself what it is that you'd like to manifest.

These principles involve knowing that there's a Higher Part of yourself than just the Ego and having a trust in your ability to be able to manifest. You must have a knowing within yourself that you are not different or separate from that which it is that you would like to be able to bring into your life. We all share the same energy and everything in the universe has an energy that flows through it

(Chi, Life Force etc.) including you and I. I believe in chiropractic you use the term Innate Intelligence.

What it boils down to is a matter of connecting yourself to these various things in the universe that you'd like to be able to create. It's really you participating in the act of creating your own mindset. Now, unconsciously, I've been doing that all of my life.

When I was a young boy, I'd put my mind to what it is that I really wanted to have. A lot of my friends would find themselves getting sick or getting colds and very often I could remember as a young boy making a decision that I wasn't going to be subjected to these kinds of things in my life. I wasn't going to get colds, talk to other people about it or complain about it. It was an inner game that I played with myself and it's a game you can play and teach to the people you care for.

Whenever I felt a sniffle coming on, rather than giving in to it, I'd connect to the ability that I believe is in myself and all other things, to heal myself. I then used to practice this sort of thing with things like prosperity and attracting things to myself. I was the only kid in the orphanage that ever had any money because I'd attract it to myself. I had an abundance mentality and the others had more of a poverty mindset.

I developed a prosperity consciousness early on and a sense of abundance about myself that I used to go out and earn money. When we had snowfalls out there in Michigan, I'd go and shovel at six in the morning without even knocking on doors. I'd go around later to tell them it was me and collect the money. I'd practice lending this money out to the other kids in the orphanage with interest rates. I learned these things, not because someone came around and told me, rather I had an intuitive knowing that I was much more powerful in my ability to create things.

I was ten years old and used to watch the Tonight Show when Steve Allen was the host (when my mother got us back together again) and I'd tell my mom that I'd be on the show one day. Sure enough, some twenty years later, the first time I did the tonight Show with Johnny Carson, Steve Allen was the very first guest.

It's not a matter of just having a positive thought, an affirmation, or a mantra. All of those are useful and important. What I'm referring to is having a knowing and then projecting that kind of energy out. Along with this you must also have the intention that goes with it and then follow through with it.

Vision

In order to have a clear, concise, and compelling vision, you must first have a nourishing of the soul and you really have to understand your own adult development. An adult has four stages of development that they generally go through according to Karl Jung in his book, **Modern Man In Search Of A Soul**, which he wrote back in the 1950's.

He said that the four stages that we go through are defined this way: The first (lowest) stage is the stage of the **ATHLETE**, which is the time in your adult life where your primary motivation and identification is with your physical appearance. How fast you can run, how you look, how attractive you are and so on. This is not a put-down of athletics, it's just what he called it.

The second stage is what he called the stage of the **WARRIOR**, which is the stage of the Ego. This is the time in your life when you take your physical bodies out into the world and really believe that they are separate from everyone and everything else. You feel the need to conquer as a warrior and you put your attention on your own quotas. What's in it for me, who can I defeat, and how much more can I get from others I perceive as being separate from me, are the questions of the day.

If you happen to get there in your lifetime, the third stage of adult development is what Jung called the stage of the **STATESMAN**. This is the time in your life when you stop asking, "What are my own quotas?" and begin to say, "What are yours?" You slowly shift from a vision of self-interest into service. You focus on the question - how may I better serve, which becomes your Mantra. Your attention is off of yourself, no longer being self-absorbed. This is where freedom and true vision begins to take shape along with a higher sense of being. In this new realm is a place you're able to find your freedom, happiness, and fulfillment

The 8 Laws of Chiropractic Success

in the service of others. When you do this, more things come to you then when you're chasing after them for yourself.

The fourth and highest stage is the stage of the **SPIRITUALIST** and this is the time when you recognize that you no longer are any of these previous three and that this world is not your home. As Jesus Christ said, "We are in this world, we are not of this world, what we are is a witness to this world." When you become a spiritual being, you become the person, not which you notice, rather you become the "noticer."

What you notice is all the stuff around you; your body, bank account, family, and all of these things. You become that which is observing those as the **SPIRITUALIST**. You have to learn to, what I call in **Your Sacred Self**, "cultivate the witness," which is learning how to witness your life rather than identifying with it.

Those are the spiritual kinds of journey's that most of us are on. Unfortunately, most people don't get to that highest level and they have to keep coming back here until they do.

Intention

Well, I think the chiropractor and chiropractic student must first understanding some essentials of healing before they delve into what their intention is to be. If you already are a chiropractor or you are going to school to learn to become one, the process of healing really involves having a knowing within yourself that someone that comes to you who's in a state of dis-repair, that you can help this person to heal. That knowing that you have has to be stronger than the knowing that the patient has that they can't heal themselves. When you have that kind of a knowing you generate an energy between yourself and the person that is seeking your help.

It is really a gaining within yourself coupled with a banishment of all doubt about your ability to heal and understand that doctors do not heal patients. If you cut yourself and a wound opens up, that wound will close all by itself quite quickly to avoid infection. The body amazingly seems to know how to do this on its own. In this sense, the body is the hero, if you will.

The great healers are the ones who convey to people, "There is an energy that exists between us of which I have a knowing and am absolutely, totally and completely certain, without any doubt at all, that I can be of help to you in healing yourself." When you are able to convey this message with that intention, it comes across with such power and strength, that the people who come to you will never doubt it. You must spend time working with your thought forms by going within and developing an appreciation and understanding of what it takes for people to heal.

You want to be able to generate that kind of healing energy which must first begin with yourself and absolutely have a knowing that you can heal you. If you have a cold, don't go around complaining about it and generating that type of energy. Rather, go to work on changing the Life Force within you. The more that you can do that within yourself and project that kind of energy, the more that when someone comes to you, you can help them heal because you are able to convince them that you absolutely know that you can be of help or assistance to them.

Service

Service can only occur when one is living in the present moment. We cannot serve in the past or in the future, only the present. Yet, the past and future are where most people spend the great majority of their time. Because of this, true service is not what's being delivered; it's something else entirely. It is the conditioning process that most people have been in, being trained by well-meaning Ego's and you become those Ego's yourselves. When you become completely and totally immersed in the present moment, what happens is you lose your mind and people are afraid to do that. They are ruled by the mind which really gropes around kind of a darkness.

When you meditate, for example, and you let go of all of your thoughts about what's going to happen in the future and all of your thoughts about what has happened in the past and immerse yourself totally in this present moment, that's when you get to know God. The Ego is terrified of you knowing God and God

The 8 Laws of Chiropractic Success

makes his appearance literally in the silence. This is what most people are terrified of because in that silence, they will come to know the Divine part of themselves, which is the only part of you that can be of service to others.

Now, everyone is always in the present moment. The question is, "How do you use up your present moment?" Do you use up your present moment commiserating with yourself or others about the past? This is called guilt. We've been trained and raised on guilt to feel bad about what you did or didn't do or to put yourself down, so you can use up your present moments constantly going over all that you should or should not have done.

You can also be using up your present moments anticipating what is going to happen and this is called worry. Using up your present moments to worry is another way of avoiding the higher part of yourself in the present moment. One of my teachers told me, "It makes no sense to worry about the things you have no control over because if you have no control over them it makes no sense to worry about them." He also said, "It makes no sense to worry about the things you do have control over because if you do have control over them it makes no sense to worry about them." So there goes everything that's possible to worry about, and yet people continue to practice this because they've been raised by similar people. So if most people are worrying most of the time, and you are either in the past or future, how can you be of adequate service to yourself let alone others?

One of the things you have to do, and I talk about in **Your Sacred Self**, is you have to erase your past. The real issue is how you are using up the present moment and not whether or not you're in it. It's really our consciousness and as Buddha says, "Do not gather, do not store." That is, do not take all of the stuff from your past and bring it into you and put labels on yourself. Understand that, "When you label me, you negate me."

What you have to do is rid yourself of all of these labels (I'm a man, woman, conservative, liberal, black/white, chiropractor, MD, republican etc.) and see yourself as a Divine spiritual essence who is here to be of service to others. You and I just happen to be in this physical body and ought to strive to have no attachment to it; knowing that who you are is not that which is constantly changing but is the part of you that never changes. That is in a different dimension altogether.

Rejection

Obstacles are judgements of the mind and it just depends on how you look at them. It's my view that we show up here on this planet for a purpose and that there are no accidents in the universe. It is a divine universe and an intelligent organism that we and the planet are a unique part of. We aren't really an organism in an environment as much as we are an organism environment. In other words, you cannot describe yourself without describing your environment and you cannot have an intelligent organism out of a stupid environment.

So if I were to describe myself walking across the floor, for example, I cannot describe myself walking without describing the floor. If you think of yourself as intelligence, you have to also think of yourself in an intelligent environment. This is how I tend to view myself and all the things that happen to me. Looking at things this way there really is no rejection, just opportunities at creation and manifestation.

Before I wrote this book called **Your Sacred Self**, I read the Kabala and some of the great spiritual literature including the New Testament and A Course In Miracles. One of the things that the Bhagavad Gita said is that we show up here for a reason. In order to be able to move from being a physical being (human being) having a spiritual experience, to a higher place which is to become a spiritual being having a human experience, you have to generate an enormous amount of energy.

Energy is a very powerful force that you have to come to grips with in your life. Everything is energy and everything is vibrating. In order to be able to generate the energy to move from being a physical being to becoming a spiritual being you must first experience a fall! All the falls of our lives (illnesses, bankruptcies,

The 8 Laws of Chiropractic Success

rejections, and break-ups etc.) are really nothing more than ways to generate energy to get yourself to a higher place. The purpose of the chiropractic adjustment in its purest form is to remove blockages from the person in order to free them up where they are able to generate this energy in order to go higher into their self-expression.

With all the falls I encounter I ask myself, "What is the lesson in this?" All the spiritual advances in our lives are generally preceded by a fall of some kind or another. So, to the metaphysical sense in which I am speaking, there are truly no obstacles or rejections — just opportunities!

Love

I've written a book called **Your Sacred Self** and when I toured the country and I asked, "What is sacred?" the answers always had to do with religion. Very few people said, "I am sacred." That is what I think is the most sacred of all, your own humanity and self-love. I think that all of us are nothing more than extensions of God. In the New Testament, in the Philippians II in verses five and six, St. Paul says, "Have in you the same mind as Christ Jesus who being in the form of God did not consider it robbery to be equal with God." Later on in St. John, Jesus says, "Know Ye, that Ye are God."

You must understand that God is not something like a big boss out there in charge of everything, keeping track of all things, and ready to punish you for any of your sins. Rather, God is the universal force that flows through all things and you are a piece of and extension of God. The God force that is in all things is also in you and that, you have to treat as sacred. When you embrace, understand, and develop these concepts, love will be apparent and ever-present in your life and practice.

Giving

One of the reasons people are not good givers is because they have not yet learned the fundamentals of receiving. We can attribute this oftentimes to the multitude of reasons that people do not heal in their lives; being bonded to the wounds of their childhood.

The 8 Laws of Chiropractic Success

You see, your biography becomes your biology and it's something to really remember in chiropractic especially. When you start looking at somebody's biology, that is their body, you don't have to go very far to find their biography. In their biography, they have all of the wounds of their past. They've come up with this idea that they were entitled to have a perfect childhood. Since they didn't and because of all the things that happened to them, they subsequently hold on to those things. They use this language of "woundology" to gain power over other people and to gain attention, pity, and so on.

One way you can give to people is by teaching them how to let go of all of those past wounds and understand that by carrying them around in their consciousness, they are embedded in the cells of their being. It is paramount to help them understand that if they want to change their health and heal, they have to allow you to assist them in ridding all of those toxic thoughts that create that negative energy and negative Life Force within them in the first place.

Chiropractic gives people an opportunity to help them heal themselves and rid themselves of the parts of their biography that are contributing to the dis-ease in their biology.

Action

Who you are is not this body that is deteriorating. Who you are is that which is observing that and noticing that. Action, the cause of all things in the physical world, is really rooted in the spiritual world. The fact that your body is aging or that an acorn becomes an oak tree, the tree-ness is not inside an acorn. You'll never find a tree-ness or anything resembling a tree in an acorn. What you know is that an acorn has the invisible, Divine Life Force within it that you can never see, touch, or get a hold of to create the physical world. And most of us, when we're in the physical world, we've lost our ability to oscillate back and forth between the material world that we notice and that which causes it; the cause of the physical world.

Once you learn to get into that non-material un-seen world (You can get there through meditation practices), you can become a co-creator in your own life and health. You have to treat that as

The 8 Laws of Chiropractic Success

sacred action and you have to see that who you are has an invisible God-Force within and is absolutely sacred; the cause of all things in the universe. Once you know that you are connected to all things and treat that as sacred, then you behave as if the God in all life really matters. You treat everything and everyone as sacred.

> What if you slept? And what if,
> in your sleep you dreamed?
> And what if, in your dream,
> you went to heaven and there
> plucked a strange and beautiful
> flower? And what if when you
> awoke, you had the flower in
> your hand?
>
> — *Samuel Taylor Coleridge*

Introduction

*"Let the beauty of what you love be
what you do." – Rumi*

When I wrote Chiropractic Revealed in 2008 and published it in 2009 I had every intention of releasing this volume, The 8 Laws of Chiropractic Success, in 2010. As we all know, life does not always go accordingly to our plans. Often times there is another force at work that has us do things according to IT'S plan. In chiropractic, we commonly refer to this force as Innate Intelligence. And for me, Innate certainly had other plans, which put this book on hold – until now, at the right place, and in the right time just about 9 years later.

I spent the greater parts of 2009-2011 promoting Chiropractic Revealed and operating a few chiropractic offices I was involved in and a part owner of in Atlanta, GA. I also was planning a large chiropractic seminar to be held in the upper gymnasium at Life University, my great alma mater. I put on "The Optimum Life Experience" in May of 2010, which had several of the speakers at the event featured in **Chiropractic Revealed**. It was a high-energy one-day event that had over 400 chiropractors, staff, and students in attendance. It was a huge success that left attendees pumped up and motivated to make a great difference in their practices, communities, their own lives, and lives of others.

In 2012 I received a message from that voice within that said, "It's time to wrap up your chiropractic practice and building-chiropractic-clinics-life and bring the next generation of students into chiropractic college." So I managed to arrange things and landed a position at Life Chiropractic College West as a new student recruiter and ultimately the Director of Recruitment. We took the college from roughly 265 students in 2012 to 650 in 2018.

When I was traveling and bringing students into chiropractic college I marveled at how few college and university students were even considering chiropractic as a career option. Their pre-health advisors mostly did not even bring it up to them as an option. Most students were looking either at PT, OT, PA, RN, or MD. They have no idea who we are and what we do because no one is telling them and therefore they're not interested in pursuing chiropractic.

They're not interested not because they don't like chiropractic. They're not interested because they DON'T KNOW. If it is to be it is up to WE! We are the ones who will turn the tide collectively and put chiropractic on the map. In our chiropractic offices we must find the diamonds in the rough and the needles in the haystack and send them to our chiropractic colleges for an open house weekend so they can get the real picture and have chiropractic as a career option. As chiropractors, take one day a month, and speak at colleges and universities in your area in their kinesiology and exercise science classes, letting the students know about this miraculous option from your positive point of view.

In 2018 that voice within spoke again (this time loudly) and said, "It is time to move on from your position at Life West and bring the book, **The 8 Laws of Chiropractic Success** off the backburner and into the hands of chiropractors, chiropractic students, and prospective chiropractic students, so they all can experience more success in their practices, future practices, and most importantly their Life." I had an amazing run traveling the USA and Internationally, bringing hundreds of new students into the chiropractic profession and making many great friends, in it and outside of it, as well. I will continue sending students to chiropractic colleges (we certainly need more chiropractors in the world) while continuing to realize some unfinished personal and entrepreneurial dreams of my own; Things that will take my full time and attention to better humanity, the planet, and the universe.

For starters, this book, **The 8 Laws of Chiropractic Success**, has a second title when you position the number 8 on its side. That title is **The ∞ Laws of Chiropractic Success** or **The Infinite Laws of Chiropractic Success**. When a chiropractor touches the spine, with the appropriate intention and whether they realize it or not, they enter into a gateway of infinite consciousness, intelligence, and wisdom, providing an opportunity for the person whom they are touching to enter the same along with them. It is through this chiropractic adjustment that both chiropractor and practice member enter the Infinite; where true healing and transformation resides.

Let's digress for a moment. When I was a chiropractic student, I was infatuated and enamored with the philosophy of chiropractic, which is also the philosophy of Life itself. Chiropractic, I understood, operated within and without the natural laws of the universe. I soaked up all I could at Life Chiropractic College (now Life University) in Marietta, GA from 1992-1996, and was literally lit-up every time I stepped foot on campus. I was fortunate to have Dr. Sid Williams at the helm and in his prime while I was there. I made it my mission as a student to see him one on one as much as I could and we'd even "run into" each other off campus at restaurants and other events. We were two like-minded souls on a ship called ChiropracTIC, bringing the Lasting Purpose; To Give, To Love, To Serve, and To Do to everyone crossing our paths and never looking for anything in return.

I wrote for the student newspaper Elan Vital during my time at chiropractic college. I interviewed many prominent chiropractors and these interviews got published in that student newspaper. One of the interviews was with a quite elderly chiropractor who knew someone that knew D.D. Palmer. I was so intrigued that I actually tracked this person down (who was well over 90 at that time) and met with him in Chicago, IL on one of my early breaks from classes.

We met at a park one cold morning, sipped hot tea, and played chess for hours. We didn't say much to one another and in fact the only words I remember that came out of my mouth

The 8 Laws of Chiropractic Success

were hello and my name. Chess was the matter at hand (he won every match) and when we were finished, or when he finished me off, he said, "Let's go for a little walk." I marveled at how energetic he was and how graceful his gate. He later told me that he'd been receiving chiropractic adjustments from birth through his nineties.

We walked many city blocks and he spoke about his encounters with D.D. Palmer, D.C. as a youth and into his early teenage years. He recalled how obsessed D.D. was with Chiropractic (he thought of nothing else) and how badly his son B.J. wanted to grow the profession into more of a well-known and mainstream entity, whereas his father often spoke about making the profession a religion and into something where people could gather for hours and talk about the Laws of Life, Infinite Intelligence, Innate Intelligence, Universal Intelligence, Spiritual concepts and matters; something modeled after the Spiritualist movement he was involved in, in the late 1800's. This gentleman also told me of how D.D. and B.J. were at terrible odds regarding their separate differing views about where the profession ought to go and how this split them up and eventually drove D.D. west where his health, both physically and mentally, diminished.

My new "old friend" and I continued to stroll the windy streets of Chicago and before we parted ways he told me that even though D.D. and B.J. were at odds, each respected the other; D.D. for how B.J. had grown Palmer College and B.J. for how his father started the profession. He continued by sharing that B.J. was an inventor and had a keen business mind, while his father was a dreamer, spiritualist, and lover of all things natural, including an enormous spine collection (both human and animal which he saw on occasion). Being at odds, he said, was almost inevitable but in the end they each played an enormous role in what we're left with today.

The last thing he said to me was to never let the flame completely burn out and that it was D.D.'s wish that every man, woman, and child on the planet have access to pure, principled, subluxation-based chiropractic care.

So here we are in 2018 and like father D.D. and son B.J. the profession is still split and at odds. What remains though are the same Universal Laws that were here before D.D. discovered chiropractic and that will be here when each of us is long gone. Let's do everything we can individually and collectively to raise this torch of light called chiropractic so in the darkness we may light the way for the masses to see their light and healing potential from within; their human potential that comes from above, down, inside, out.

It has recently been said that we are the entire universe manifesting through a human nervous system. Therefore, we are all intricately connected to all there is and all there is not. We are holographic in nature and mirror images of the universe itself. Let's gather together and remember the words of Alan Cohen, "The dance is never done and the song is never sung until the love of the truth has made us ONE." The love of the truth in chiropractic shall set us and the world free. That is the ultimate success we can experience. There are many more people not under chiropractic care in the world than there are. It is up to each of us to spread its glorious messages to the masses; for it is there within them that the beauty, essence, truth, and value of chiropractic can be found.

May you now sit back, relax, and enjoy this compilation of fascinating facts, spectacular stories, mystical messages, and wondrous wisdom, from some of the greatest in the chiropractic profession, aimed to propel you higher and to experience massive success in chiropractic practice and Life.

I give to you, with Love —The 8 Laws of Chiropractic Success.

— *David K. Scheiner, D.C.*

Chapter 1

"You have to be willing to allow the person you are today to DIE so that you can give birth to the person you are meant to become." — Les Brown

Law One – Mindset

David K. Scheiner, D.C.

Mindset is similar to the thermostat in your home. You can set it to cool, warm, hot, fan only or completely off. Our minds are similar in that, like the thermostat, we control them. Are you going to upload negative doom and gloom thoughts? Or will you program your minds for happiness, joy, success, and fulfillment?

We hear it time and time again, "We are what we think about all day long," and "What we think about we bring about." Thoughts really are things – delicate things – and our mindset is a direct reflection of the station you tune it in to. What are you programming your mind with? I said long ago, "Having an attitude of gratitude determines your longitude and latitude in life." Ask yourself, "What results, if accomplished, would be worth the necessary time and efforts in getting them?"

You're familiar with the comparison between two chiropractors practicing across the street from one another. One complains that there's too many chiropractors in the town and the other across the street merely has time to talk because their reception room is filled, as is each of their adjusting tables – all day long! If these chiropractors switched offices, within thirty days the slow practice will be booming and the busy practice will be a ghost town. Why? Because of mindset. B.J. Palmer once said, "When you get the BIG idea all else follows." When you set your mind right (and only you can do that) all else follows.

Just allow yourself to be and to stop trying and doing. Set your mind towards gratitude and open up your heart. Even though you know that you can do, sometimes it's just as important to let it be and not do what you always do. In fact, try mixing it up for a while. Take a different route to school or work. Rearrange the furniture in your office or home. Take a different cardio class at the gym and introduce some new foods into your eating habits.

In order to create the space for something new to emerge we must first get to know our own mind before we can truly set-mind-right. Get in touch and work with your subconscious mind (our filter of sanity) and become familiar with where your fears congregate. Once you get to know those and work on them you'll enter into a sacred place where a new mindset will automatically emerge and your life will take on a wonderfully positive new shape, filled with hope, abundance, success, and joy.

When you are chosen to be a chiropractor, an entire new realm of possibility is brought into your life. It's the road less traveled, where you get to blaze a new path in a unique way and where something wonderful comes to be. Something new, unseen before, and not from the past. Becoming a chiropractor opens for each of you a realm of possibility to bring a new world into existence from nothing. Inside that realm of possibility is a blank canvas where all possibilities reside. You literally get to choose how you want your life and mindset to be.

Frederick A. Schofield, D.C.

Sun Tzu said, *"If you know your enemies and know yourself, you will not be imperiled in 100 battles; if you do not know your enemies but do know yourself, you will win one and lose one; if* *you do not know your enemies or know yourself, you will be imperiled in every single battle."*

Before I guide you into creating new possibilities for your Life and Practice, let's take a moment to understand the Mindset.

You run your SuperComputer, your Brain, which runs your thinking, feeling, and acting.

You are in charge. You are in charge of your motivation. You are in charge of your persuasion skills. You are in charge of your self-esteem, self-image, and self-awareness. You are in charge of the memory of your experiences both negative and positive. You are in charge of your mindset.

You have the ability to change your thoughts, feelings, and actions AND when and how you De-Sire it.

Remember the words of Alfred Korzybski, "The map is not the territory." Your mindset is made up of maps of pictures of your experiences, perspectives, awareness, and your emotions. You have the ability and resources to take action despite your positive or negative memory.

Your Mindset is the direction in which you act. You have 2 Mindsets: constructive mindset or destructive mindset. Constructive mindset moves you towards constructive motives and moves you away from Destructive mindset. For instance you grew up NOT having money. So you decide that the rest of your life you are going to **Your Mindset is the direction in which you act.** move away from that destructive picture of no money. We call that destructive mindset. Your motivation may be to create the most amazing practice serving thousands of patients and you are looking forward to that prosperity in practice. We call that constructive mindset. Be careful of destructive mindset because you will not enjoy this Mindset twenty years later in Practice. I was raised in Africa. My Father used to say, "Get a Job!" and "You Think Money Grows On Trees?" All of these are short-term, destructive mindsets.

Turn your mindset around towards a constructive mindset.

The 8 Laws of Chiropractic Success

Remember your motivation is your Mindset.

Affirm:

> *Divine Order Radiates thru my Practice*
> *I Live in Divine Prosperity and Attract Double*
> *Digit New Patients*
> *Divine Prosperity Radiates Thru My Affairs*

Stay in a constructive Mindset versus a destructive Mindset. Go To Work Every day!!! And we will See You at the Top!!! Be Still and Sow and SO IT IS!!!

Billy DeMoss, D.C.

Mindset is a your attitude in life. There's no doubt that having a positive, optimistic, and happy attitude goes way further than having a pessimistic attitude. If you feel positive about your contributions towards others and towards the planet, you're going to have a greater impact — "Using honey to attract bees," as the saying goes.

I'm not perfect when it comes to optimism. I get frustrated about certain conditions that are prevalent in today's society like vaccinations, pollution, and the degradation of our oceans. Then again, I come back to being positive about human beings being smart enough to solve these problems. The youth of today make me super optimistic about change and progress in our profession and our world. My positivity influences my success because it allows me to care for myself and others.

I take breaks regularly and recharge with vacations through-out the year, which is something I recommend you do too. I've found that success follows when you take care of yourself and don't get too worn out. Be happy, be grateful, be positive, be nice to others, and do things for the right reasons. It's never about you — it's about how you contribute to others and the planet.

Guy Riekeman, D.C.

You must understand in the depths of your minds that you are the leaders and you have to get on leading your flock. You have to do your homework and know what it is that you're leading. You need to do your homework and make the determination to live the life you really want to live.

Otherwise, you may end up getting shocked into re-evaluating your life because of a trauma. Maybe your business goes under or you lose a child. Something happens where, all of a sudden, you say, "I have to live my life differently." There's nothing to lose because you have lost everything at that point. For some people, this is the only time they'll be able or willing to change. But, if you want to do it more rationally, you need a coach to walk you through the process.

Chuck Ribley, D.C.

How I think is the backdrop of creating my life.

Universal Intelligence is in all matter and continually gives to it ALL its properties and actions, thus maintaining it in existence.

Innate Intelligence is an individualized expression of Universal Intelligence in living man.

The POWER that made the body, Heals the body.

These statements are a validation of what I believe. We create our life from our beliefs.

The thoughts that I think repeatedly with fire, passion, and emotion become beliefs and enter into the quantum field of unlimited possibilities, which create my world.

From this foundation of beliefs, I have a foundation that supports my ability to enter into a world of healing by adjusting vertebral subluxation, enabling Innate to restore life and health.

My beliefs also support my ability to affect the quantum field for the success of my chiropractic practice and also my internal and external worlds.

The 8 Laws of Chiropractic Success

Donny Epstein, D.C.

Mindset is a result of the amount of energy available for Innate Intelligence to organize the Educated or conditioned mind. I prefer the concept of a Mind UN-set and present. A set mind represents a finite amount of energy to match one's desires or focus and/or achieve certain goals. Rather than using any Set mental focus to connect to the practice member, being present and allowing whatever mindset emerges better serves the practice member as a being or soul — and not simply a role.

Everything we consider real is fueled by energy and expressed as Intelligence. Around all energy is a field of information. We respond to this primary field. Consciousness represents information that is observed. When we are present with a person there is an entrainment or attunement with their field. This changes both our mindset and theirs and liberates available energy. This increased energy between us and those we serve, enhances our focus, what we observe, and the care we give.

The heightened energy associated with presence fuels Innate Intelligence's manifestation.

As energy is lost from a system, the expression of the intelligence is compromised. Form, emotion, and thought can no longer exist in their prior state. Collapsing to a lower functional level, entropy sets in. In contrast, as more available energy is added to a system it evolves to a higher order. Each mindset or level of presence perfectly represents a precise level of energy. Presence energetically impacts all of our relationships and enhances the innate response.

With presence and an elevated and flexible mindset, there is more available coherent energy in the field between you and your practice member. This energizes what is possible when you are speaking with them, analyzing their spine and information systems, and adjusting them.

So, from what I call an EpiEnergetics perspective (EpiEnergetics is the conscious and ecological use of energy and information is to produce the extraordinary), mindset and presence are really reflections of one's Energy Level with its appropriate expression of Innate Intelligence, fueling the Educated (conditioned) Intelligence.

It is imperative that you always view at least two perspectives simultaneously. This activates the more complex thinking mind and helps nurture presence allowing us to ask, "How will I best collaborate with this person to OPTIMIZE his or her higher Innate expression? How can this adjustment impact this person's life and the field of humanity even more; consistent with his or her true nature?"

The Australian Spinal Research Foundation's definition of vertebral subluxation considers the loss of being and of coherence (energy efficiency) along with the structural, neurological, and functional changes.

If you add any of these three simultaneous perspectives you can activate the "spiritual" or post rational mind to engage a higher order response. I encourage you to consider beingness and coherence as vital parts of your evolving mindset and increasing presence with the knowing that the other factors are already in your awareness. With practice you will suddenly and effortlessly invoke what is true beyond the educated mind, both yours and your practice member's, and increase the energetic efficiency of your beingness, your interactions, and the care you deliver.

Cathy Wendland-Colby, D.C.

The epigram: "Your attitude, more than your aptitude, determines your altitude," spoke to me as I began walking the halls during first quarter of pre-requisites at Life Chiropractic College. This epigram did more than reinforce the belief my parents instilled in us that mindset was important. It drove home the point that Mindset is Everything!

The vast majority of people you meet have let the world beat them down. They've bought into the marketing schemes that repeatedly convinced them their bodies aren't sexy enough, faces aren't pretty enough, and that health is only available by prescription. Trusting little children believed their parents, teachers, and peers who constantly pointed out every flaw and failure while telling them they were bad, stupid, ugly, unpopular...and worse. And like kudzu, with its ever-invasive vines, the roots run so deep that no matter how many times you try to clear that negativity, even in adults, it just keeps creeping back up.

Changing your stinking thinking isn't easy because you must first recognize that while others were wrong for what they said, at some point you believed their words enough to incorporate them into your inner dialogue.

You must acknowledge this in order to accept responsibility for your inner dialogue from this moment forward and rightfully claim your power. You are strong enough, smart enough, bold enough, and yes worthy enough. You are enough. You are more than enough.

Set your mind before you start your day, refocus at every challenge, and program your inner dialogue before bed with the words and thoughts necessary to manifest your ideal life.

Whatever goals you set for yourself, whether you think you can or think you can't, either way you're right. Every action, outcome, and product began as a whisper in the corners of one's mind — be watchful of what you allow in.

Where some wander haphazardly through life, those with a made-up mind walk confidently in the direction of their success. The best part is - you get to choose your mindset at every moment. The right mindset nails an exclamation point where others before you hung a question mark.

John Demartini, D.C.

The one major thing that has doctors and students realize their true practice potential is a value system. One of my clients, a Midwest doctor, said he had been in practice for a number of years but had always just gotten by with minimal income. We looked at and identified his values and it was obvious that he set a high value on metaphysics, on going to classes, seminars, and personal development lectures. He also put a high value on his wife and kids and wanted a comfortable life.

He was making just enough money to do all the things he wanted to do. He didn't need a big practice to reach his modest goals, so he had a modest practice.

Then his wife said, "We've been married for years and I really expected a greater lifestyle and if you aren't going to provide that, I'm moving on." All of a sudden he had this wake-up call that he was either going to lose his wife and kids or he was going to have to get into gear.

That automatically shifted his values to some degree. He came for a consultation and I showed him how to place his practice, income, and wealth higher on his list of values and how to integrate his metaphysical beliefs into his practice and experience fulfillment.

You may need to reorganize your value system to such a degree that your practice and life shift. When you shift your values, you shift your life.

∞

Amanda and Jeremy Hess, D.C.'s

A friend of ours, Ronnie Doss, always says, "If you can learn to master the moment, you can learn to master your life." We really believe that mindset resides in the moment. Life is made up of moments and the hardest part of keeping the right mindset in life is when you don't feel like it!

The key to mindset and maintaining forward motion in life and in chiropractic is to *act your way* into a feeling and doing the things you know you should be doing. So many times in life, when we know we should be doing something that will propel ourselves or our practice forward, we simply don't feel like it! How many times have we thought about going in the office early to get prepared for a big day or get the team fired up or get a new promotion going, but we don't follow through with it! All of us are victim, at one time or another, of not feeling like we should exercise (our body or mind), when we know we should.

The important thing to remember about mindset is doing the right things at the right time. The way to control your mindset is to be able to control your actions and let the right mindset and actions rule your life; not your feelings! We need to "Act our way into a Feeling" in many cases, and as we start the action of doing something, the feeling will soon follow. For example, if you've ever started to exercise when you didn't feel like it, you have experienced during or after the exercise how good you feel, even though you didn't start out that way.

Mindset is also heavily dictated by who you allow to speak into your life, what you listen to, who you spend time with, and what you choose to read. Mindset is what Earl Nightingale referred to in his classic book as, "The Strangest Secret." Earl talks about, and proves that, "We become what we think about," and he uses the analogy of a farmer sowing seeds of a poisonous plant and that of corn in a field, likening it to the mind.

The Mind doesn't care what you sow. Be careful of what your input is, as it can affect your output. Our mindset, or what we choose to sow, or focus on, or think about, becomes our reality. All of us have been beaten down, suffered failures, and have insecurities from our past, BUT we must take the time to start sowing and thinking-on the right things, shifting our mindset to one of success, abundance, and being the person who will make a positive difference in the lives of those coming into our practice to receive chiropractic care.

D.D. Humber, D.C.

Your mindset is key to your success and this is certainly true for the Chiropractor and the Chiropractic student. First of all, Chiropractic can be very challenging for the student. It requires two to four years pre-requisite classes and then almost another four years for a D.C. Degree. This takes a lot of study, will, and determination.

The 8 Laws of Chiropractic Success

As for me, the decision to become a Chiropractor was easy. Two older brothers were already D.C.'s and I had been helped greatly with health issues from the early age of thirteen. There's no question this experience helped me greatly in making my decision to become a Chiropractor.

Being a successful D.C. begins with knowing without any doubt that Chiropractic works. That, my friend, is having a made-up mind, without which success cannot be assured. Dr. Sid Williams, Founder and President of Life Chiropractic College (now Life University) used to illustrate this by "the dropping of the keys," thus proving that Chiropractic works like the law of gravity. The keys — once dropped — will **always** fall down. Chiropractic **always** works when the right adjustment is given — not some of the time, but every time. Having this understanding and acceptance of Chiropractic gives one the mindset needed to become a successful D.C.

Jessica Harden, D.C.

Mindset is one of the most fundamental and most overlooked tools for success. It is more than just a positive attitude. It is our interpretation of our environment and our self-reflection within it. Ronnie Doss, a leadership coach who dives into how we perceive our world, discusses the concepts of Fact versus Meaning. Facts are the events in our life and the meaning is our interpretation of those events. For instance, consider graduation from chiropractic school. Some will say graduation meant freedom and excitement. To others, it meant anxiety and tearful goodbyes. Both sets of individuals walk across the same stage and hear the same speeches so why would some see this event as a joyful occasion and others recall an anxious turning point? It is because these two groups have assigned different meanings to the same event and those meanings will create different emotions and different experiences.

It is often said that your mind can make you or break you.

The 8 Laws of Chiropractic Success

By examining the impact of these meanings you assign, you'll discover this to be true. What if you had a delay in getting a building permit for your first office? Some would say this would be inconvenient and stressful but what if you could see this as an opportunity for extra time to prepare and meet more people? What if you invested thousands of dollars into an advertising project but did not see a great return on the investment? You could see it as a waste and feel regret and another person could see it as a payment towards their entrepreneurial education and learn from it. The interpretations of these pivotal events would change how the individual acts or executes decisions in the future. What may be even more vital than your interpretation is how you view yourself in these circumstances.

Angela Duckworth, a leading psychologist studying GRIT, speaks about growth mindset; a belief that people are growth-oriented, malleable, and can learn through both experience and effort. As Duckworth puts it, "We can approach a situation, good or bad, and ask, what can I do here to change things for the better and to keep things on course?" The opposite is a fixed mindset, which is a deeply rooted belief that people are ultimately unchangeable. If you can filter these meanings you assign to life events through a growth mindset, you can transform your capacity to improve and increase your endurance to push forward towards success.

Brian Kelly, D.C.

First you need to define what success is for you. You all have different wants, needs, desires and values in life, and no two people will measure success the same way. For some people a successful life is one of balance between seeing patients three days a week and having an abundance of family time. For others it may be building a high-volume practice working six days a week.

It is known that what you think about you bring about. Any person who spends a large amount of time thinking in terms of abundance and joy, will have more of it show up in their life. If you think and focus on lack and scarcity, then this will show up too. To prove this theory, ask people who have incredible success in their lives what they think about. What do they read or not read? Who do they spend time with? You will find they spend time with those who also constantly work at developing a success mindset at a very high-level.

Is this easy? No. Does it take discipline and hard work? Yes. Is it worth it? You can experiment by trying both and then determine if it is or not. We all have the same 168 hours in a week. How you choose to spend them and who you choose to spend them with determines your entire future.

We have both a conscious and a subconscious mind. Because 95% of all thinking is in the subconscious mind and developed in our first few years of life, accessing the subconscious mind is essential for the mindset you wish to develop. Meditation is one of the most effective strategies in accomplishing this.

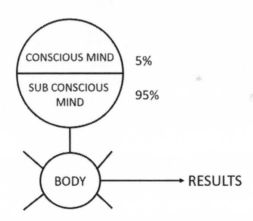

I am convinced that mindset, followed by a thoughtful and well executed plan (strategy), is the key to achieving your dreams and goals. This has helped me have significant achievement in my chiropractic career and I am now spending my time helping others who wish to achieve greatness in their chiropractic and personal lives.

The 8 Laws of Chiropractic Success

Jason Deitch, D.C.

Clearly mindset matters. As discussed in Napoleon Hill's all time classic book on success, **Think and Grow Rich**, your mindset is the "bullseye" of the target of your life. I've heard it said multiple times, "Whether you think you can or you think you can't, either way you're right." Your mindset matters in many ways and for many reasons.

Let's start with a few of the most important, such as the impact your attitude has on your experience in life, each and every day. If you have a mindset that you have to grind it out, that people don't want what you have unless their insurance pays for it, that the only thing people want is quick pain relief, that will guide your energy level, conversations, and investments of where and how you promote yourself and your practice. Your practice and your life then are a direct reflection of what you think about all day.

A mindset based on your desire to serve your community, to awaken them to a new disruptive way of thinking about health care, and your commitment to attract people interested in natural healing will drive you to have very different conversations which will impact the ways you promote yourself and your practice throughout your community. These ways of thinking and being will eventually yield great outcomes for your practice and life.

As the word "mindset" implies, it's the frequency or vibration your mind is set to. Imagine your mind working like a radio where you choose which station to dial your mind to receive and play. Some people will just let whatever station they happen to land on play-out throughout their lives. Others, on the other hand, will let other people set their mindset based on their desires, not their own. What's best for you and the people you come across is to realize the power within you to set your mind to the station of your choice.

What station do you like to be tuned into? Do you like music that makes you happy, makes you dance, talk radio that informs you or entertains you? That frequency you set your mind to; happy, enthusiastic, generous, abundant, and skilled is what will ultimately determine your success.

Arno Burnier, D.C.

What's important to include when developing your mindset are a set of clear, precise, and concise principles. You must have strong and sustaining guiding principles. I'm absolutely floored when I run into chiropractors who have been in practice fifteen or twenty years and don't even understand what healing is about or where healing comes from. That, to me, is bewildering because all they've been doing for twenty years is trying to "fix" people. Develop your mindset early on and have it guide you within or you will be left without.

Gerard Clum, D.C.

I think we often have a very unrealistic idea that most people move in the direction of logic and reasoning. On occasion they do, but more often they don't. That's why we need to relate to people on an experiential level before we start talking to them on a conceptual level.

I remember Sid Williams, D.C. talking about missionaries traveling the world. He said it's a lot easier for people to listen to your spiritual message when you've taken the wrinkles out of their bellies. Take care of their needs first and then approach them with how their needs can be better served over time with what you have to offer.

Tim Young, D.C.

Your mindset, as it relates to your success in the chiropractic profession, is greatly influenced by the environment you were raised in or the academic environment in which you studied. What I have witnessed over the past twenty-five years in this profession is that whatever mindset the individual chiropractor has in regards to what he or she can or cannot do, they are right.

The beauty of chiropractic is it allows for a self-fulfilling prophecy. There are no limits other than the ones each individual sets for themselves. You must ask yourself the question, "What do I want?" Upon the answer to that question rests your entire future.

James Sigafoose, D.C.

One major thing that keeps doctors from realizing their full potential is the education they receive. By that I mean that faith comes by hearing of the word. That's exactly what it says in the Scriptures.

So, if you keep hearing that the only thing that works is the physical application of a therapeutic model, you build faith in that and the more faith you have in that model, the more you are inclined to talk, live, and practice that way.

Conversely, if you have learned that Innate does the work, you create an entirely different mindset, one that allows you to go beyond the limitations of therapy.

Jim Dubel, D.C.

The correct mindset, or way of thinking about Chiropractic, is to know with complete certainty that Chiropractic works every time and with every patient. Once you have established this as your life and practice mantra, everything falls perfectly into place.

Every person I meet, I know that within my mind, I can change their life with a Chiropractic adjustment.

Neil Cohen, D.C.

Everyone has a mindset, yet it's what that mind is set on that matters. Mindset is defined as "The established set of attitudes held by an individual." These so called attitudes are not just relative to your success, they are intimately connected to your foundation for failure as well. Through empiricism, rationalism, and cultural norms, you will establish your own philosophy leading to a particular mindset with little regard for even its own veracity. After all, having "no philosophy" is a philosophy and a mindset in and of itself.

In order for a chiropractor and chiropractic student to be successful, you must first possess the foundation for success which is a "made up mind." Without the power of the made up mind there is the looming danger of being tossed about "to and fro" like a ship lost in a turbulent ocean storm. Your made up mind is the rudder controlled by the ship's wheel, keeping you on purpose applying and executing the strategies necessary to keep you on course.

At any moment, you are fully cognizant and keenly aware of the "definite major purpose" in your life. There is nothing that can move you off of that purpose. There is no "trying" to achieve your purpose, there's only determination and will. It is a matter of *when* I will succeed and not *if* I might succeed. Successful chiropractors and students will fail but that ought not deter you from your plan to succeed. The key is succeeding by inevitably failing forward.

Liam Schubel, D.C.

Mindset is fundamental to everything you wish to achieve and be in your lives. Most chiropractic students and chiropractors however never spend much time working on their mindset. Sadly, the value of clarity and Spizz are highly underestimated as it relates to chiropractic success. As a result we have at times a profession that is rife with apathy, low self-esteem, and desperate to settle for table scraps.

The good news is that this can be changed immediately. A decision, plan, and actions to reprogram the way you think can happen today and start producing great rewards tomorrow. You can have anything you want in this world if you are specifically clear as to what exactly that is, how long you wish to take to

The 8 Laws of Chiropractic Success

achieve it, and what sacrifices you are willing to make while taking the massive action required to obtain it. A clearly defined purpose held steadfastly in your minds-eye can provide the fuel to take the persistent action that you need to take to achieve your dreams.

Your mindset needs to be exercised daily just like your physical body. Remember that you live in a world that has an entirely different understanding of where health comes from. Dr. B.J. Palmer used to say, "Who can anchor to an unanchored mind?" You must anchor your thots in positivity, purpose, and philosophy. If you do not immerse yourself in chiropractic and develop an unbridled passion to share it with others, you run the risk of losing steam and giving up.

The most successful practitioners on the planet have absolute congruency between their mindsets and their communications. Your non-verbal communications are way more powerful than anything you will ever say to a practice member. Congruent non-verbal communication requires a solid mindset. This is not developed by accident. Rather, it is developed by choice. So choose wisely and early on in your career!

Reggie Gold, D.C.

The problem with the chiropractic mindset can be traced back to the origins of chiropractic itself. D.D. Palmer was trying to cure deafness when he adjusted Harvey Lillard. Every chiropractic adjustment given by D.D. Palmer and by B.J. Palmer was to treat and cure disease. That fits perfectly into the definition of the practice of medicine. Almost every dictionary will tell you that medicine is the diagnosis, treatment, and cure of disease as well as the prevention of disease and the maintenance of health.

That is exactly what chiropractors are trained to do. They come into chiropractic with that in mind. It is reinforced by their education. They get tested on it before they get a license to practice, and they spend their life practicing what they learned.

Then I come along and talk to them about what chiropractic

could be, what its potential is. They applaud but it goes right over their heads. They give me standing ovations but they haven't the faintest idea of what I'm talking about.

I challenge them to explain chiropractic without mentioning the words health, sickness, or cure. I tell them to call me the first time they've managed to do that. I waited my entire life for the first call. They feel they don't have the ability to change because the public demands the practice of chiropractic *health care*. People have learned that if the M.D. doesn't get them well, maybe the chiropractor will.

In fact, chiropractic really doesn't exist for the public. What they're getting is spinal manipulative therapy. The majority of chiropractors believe that spinal manipulative therapy *is* chiropractic. The idea of chiropractic without therapy just doesn't occur to them.

There may be twenty chiropractors in the whole world who understand. I'm beginning to see points of light and eventually those points of light are touching other points of light and some-day — beyond my lifetime certainly — those points of light will coalesce and set the world on fire.

Do you understand the true messages of chiropractic and are you one of those points of light?

Brad Glowaki, D.C.

Your mindset establishes your road forward.

Think at a higher level so that you can help people live at a higher level. Also, recognize that you can't think at a level higher than you feel. Equally as important is your ability to consistently be cognizant of how you feel and take the necessary steps to ensure you are feeling your best so that you can perform at your highest potential.

Continually raise your self-image and see yourself beyond what your current self-esteem allows you to feel. Having a low self-image will inhibit the results you achieve. Raise your self-image and you will ultimately raise your results.

The 8 Laws of Chiropractic Success

Claudia Anrig, D.C.

Chiropractors and students set their own mindset on what they think they can and cannot do. Some people seem to think that the day I opened up my door and put out my shingle, crowds immediately flooded into my office. Guess what? No one was waiting for me — and no one is waiting for *you*. If you think they are, you're in for a big wake-up call and you'll be eating pork and beans the rest of your life.

The day you graduate from chiropractic college, you simply receive a piece of paper. After that, you have to figure out exactly what you need to work harder at and where you have to use extra elbow grease.

It's hard work to develop a practice. It'll be easier if you get rid of the mindset that everyone is waiting for you and, instead, have a specific game plan about what will work for your personality, your community, and the demographics you want to attract. Then, strive to excel and be the best you can be!

Steve Judson, D.C.

Your mindset, which comes from the truth of who you are, is what will set you free. The mind is the engine that fuels your soul and

The mind is the engine that fuels your soul...

with your mind set on what you really want in this lifetime, anything is possible. When you know, that you know, that you know, what you really want, then you must take massive action to set the mind afire and you're never to take your eyes off the target. Your mindset will create the outcome of your life.

The beautiful thing is that you get to choose what you focus on in your mind. When you focus on massive abundance, all else will come from hard work, long days, and sleepless nights.

Gilles LaMarche, D.C.

Carol S. Dweck, Ph.D., wrote the book, Mindset — The New Psychology of Success, after years of studying human behavior. What she discovered is the power of mindset. She explains that it's not only our abilities and talents that will bring success, but whether a person approaches life with a fixed or a growth mindset. In other words, how you choose to show up as a chiropractic student or a chiropractor matters. Do you show up ready to learn and open to possibility? Are you ready to put in time, effort, and be the best version of you every moment of everyday, or do you often choose to slack off? How you show up always matters.

Converting life's setbacks is a key to experiencing future successes.

The passion for stretching yourself and sticking to it even, and especially, when it's not going particularly well, is the hallmark of a growth mindset and the seed to living a successful life long-term. We've all heard the sayings: "Nothing ventured, nothing gained" and "If at first you don't succeed, try again." Converting life's setbacks is a key to experiencing future successes.

Are you a person who believes that your personality, character, and intelligence cannot be changed, or do you believe that with time and some effort you can improve and change substantially? Having a growth mindset is all about your willingness to see possibility for improvement and when you bring the best of yourself to the forefront and persevere, you get to create the life you truly want to create.

You have an ability to develop and be great! After all, you were born to thrive; engineered for success. Show up in your life with the willingness to put in 100% effort daily and combine it with a "get'er" done attitude and enjoy what happens. Effort is what makes you smart, talented, and successful, whether in your studies, your practice, your relationships, or your health.

Remember, pessimism never won any battle and optimism (positive mindset) has led many people to amazing and exciting lives filled with accomplishments. Mindset matters.

The 8 Laws of Chiropractic Success

Daniel & Richelle Knowles, D.C.'s

Your Mindset is your most valuable Asset.

There are immutable laws and principles of success that are universal, and mindset is one at the top. It has been repeated over and over that your thoughts become things, and *where* you focus the powerful thought-receiver of your brain, impacts the channels and radio stations you'll receive transmissions from. Like the old computer term, "Garbage in, garbage out," when you tune yourself to a channel that's broadcasting garbage, you yourself are going to experience garbage.

Success requires the fertile ground of an outstanding mindset channel to be tuned in to. Consistent tune-ups to your mindset allows for the greatest and most coherent channel, which is vital to your success. In fact, it's your greatest asset.

Many people think mindset means repeating affirmations over and over. People can read, recite, and repeat affirmations all day long. However, if they're receiving signals from a garbage station, they will merely be affirming on unfertile and unproductive soil. To fertilize the soils of success, focus your inner tuner to receive the clear signals of an outstanding mindset.

Armand Rossi, D.C.

Doctors and students think of themselves the way they do because of a limited or empowering mindset. They say to themselves (and others), "I can do this. I can't do that."

My highest day in practice was 386 people but when I tell other doctors that, they immediately say, "Oh that can't be done."

Well it was done — by me! And if I can do it, it can be done by anybody. I think your own limitations keep you back more than anything else. Let go of the idea that you can ONLY do this much or you CAN'T do that. You can do anything you put your mind to!

∞

Joe Strauss, D.C.

Chiropractors and chiropractic students ought to have an evangelistic mindset and a desire to work hard to communicate to the community what chiropractic is. When you do not, people won't understand what chiropractic does and won't flock into your offices.

People have to understand what chiropractic is and have a desire for it. I always use the analogy that you could be giving away $10,000 mink coats on the street corner but if you're in a town where everyone is a member of PETA, you won't find any takers.

I think the same thing is true with chiropractic care. For two years, I had a "box on the wall" practice (where patients paid on the honor system what they could afford or what they thought my services were worth) but I was really struggling. That's because I wasn't out there talking about chiropractic, about how innate intelligence heals and runs the body. I was virtually giving chiropractic away for free but there weren't many takers until I realized I had to educate my people and community about chiropractic's uniqueness.

Christopher Kent, D.C.

What's often missing from your mindset is something Patrick Gentempo calls *The Silent Dread.* Many people are reluctant to talk about this, but it goes to the heart of the greatest challenge many chiropractors face.

The Silent Dread is the underlying fear that while you understand the potential of chiropractic, that subluxations can have a devastating effect on human health and human potential, and that the nervous system is the master system of the body, you will be unable to deliver the goods. This self-doubt is a major problem for many doctors and students.

Yet, many chiropractors have an even more serious affliction. They don't understand the true value of chiropractic in the first place, at least not in their heart of hearts. This problem surfaces most frequently among those who got into chiropractic without having first lived it or experienced its wondrous benefits.

Be honest, would you follow your recommendations and pay your fees for the services you offer? That may sound silly but think about it. If you require people to sign up for 100 visits in advance and pay up front $5,000-8,000 (or whatever the figure is) ask yourself whether you would make that commitment. If the answer is not only "yes, I would" but "YES, I am," then you are on a good path.

When patients come into your office, do you examine their insurance before you examine them? If their insurance pays for modalities, do they get modalities but if their insurance doesn't pay for modalities, then they don't? Do you think that's a good way to practice? Is that what you'd want for yourself, your spouse, child, mother, and father? If you're ever in doubt about the way you practice, apply the Golden Rule and you'll get your answer.

Ross McDonald and Rebecca Vickery, D.C.'s

When studying to be a chiropractor, we constantly hear that our community is waiting for us to show up and change it for the better. This may be the case but it takes a great deal of hard work and dedication to achieve this.

Carol Dweck coined the terms fixed and growth mindset. Having a growth mindset is key to being able to be successful. You have to roll with the blows and not dwell too much on the highs and successes. It is best to learn equally from both in order to help work out who you are, what you want, and where you wish to go with your practice and life.

Having a growth mindset and learning from your experiences will ensure that you ultimately increase your neural growth by the actions you take such as using good strategies, asking questions, and practicing with an attitude of gratitude. This can enable growth, greater achievement, and success.

The 8 Laws of Chiropractic Success

Thom Gelardi, D.C.

Your mindset must include a sense of professional mission on a level of abstraction that differentiates the chiropractic objective of practice from that of other health care professions.

A clear sense of practice objective and/or how to implement it causes a clear sense of confidence in the doctor. The doctor's clear purpose affects the office staff and practice members, resulting in a high degree of enthusiasm, retention, and referrals.

B. J. Palmer, D.C. said that you have to be a radical to move people a little bit. But you have to know what you are radical about. It has been said that the whole world steps aside for the person who knows where he or she is going.

Today, in general, there is an absence of a clear sense of chiropractic's purpose. For many, unfortunately, it is an alternative therapy. This lack of understanding is not the fault of the chiropractor, for chiropractic's intended purpose is no longer taught. Our chiropractic educational curriculum has been corrupted by small, fear-filled minds, believing that chiropractic will be accepted in proportion to its similarity to medicine.

D. D. Palmer, D.C. wrote clearly the purpose or mission of the profession he founded: "Chiropractic is a name I originated to designate the science and art of adjusting vertebrae. It does not relate to the study of etiology, or any branch of medicine. Chiropractic includes the science and art of adjusting vertebrae — the knowhow and the doing."

∞

Jeanne Ohm, D.C.

Chiropractors must incorporate in their mindset the inclusion of children in their practices. I had three major surgeries and a million health issues as a kid. When I was nineteen, a simple adjustment by a chiropractor changed all that for me. I endured years of symptoms and suffering before I got under chiropractic care.

Given the effects the birth process can have on a child's cranium, spine, and nervous system, all kids need to have their spines checked for vertebral subluxation.

The 8 Laws of Chiropractic Success

I realize some doctors are very apprehensive about working with babies but caring for children isn't difficult and you don't even need to adapt your normal technique for them. You'll be amazed at how quickly you learn to feel the different areas of resistance in a baby's spine. Granted, it requires a different level of communication — mostly non-verbal — but that is an intuitive talent that proves valuable not only with kids but when dealing with and caring for people in all areas of your life.

If you're apprehensive about checking children's spines, go to someone who does it and watch what they do or take some classes to get over that psychological hump. Pick up the baby!

CJ Mertz, D.C.

God gave each of us three gifts: time, energy, and focus — what I call "TEF." Your mindset comes from an understanding of how to truly manage time, which is the first huge stumbling block to hurdle. The second is your level of energy, which is going to affect your mindset in a wild way. Finally, there's the ability to sustain correct focus.

These three things work together just like mind, body, and spirit. You can't really separate them since they're so intertwined.

The quality of your life and practice boils down to the caliber of your TEF. If you have a relatively undisciplined lifestyle — you go to bed too late, don't wake up on time, don't set aside time to pray, meditate, stretch, exercise, or feed your mind with right thoughts that sustain right focus throughout the day — your TEF is going to be adversely affected.

Compare the TEF of a chiropractor who has more than a 1,000 patient visits a week with the TEF of a doctor who sees 100 or so. It's night and day. The glorious thing is that you can improve your TEF. It's all about managing time, increasing energy, and sustaining focus. When you can do those three things, you can have the mindset that allows you to reach unlimited heights!

The 8 Laws of Chiropractic Success

Janice Hughes, D.C.

YOUR Mindset is the most powerful tool and weapon that you have. It can be sharpened and honed for good, and/or can be the negative or limiting factor in your entire life. Paraphrasing author Maxwell Maltz, the mind does not know the difference between something real versus something perceived in explicit detail. This means that your mindset, your own thinking, has more to do with your success as a Chiropractor or DC2B than any of the concrete actions you are taking.

I use the simple mantra — Thoughts Become Things! What we think we attract and create in our life. What you choose to focus on, becomes your 'reality'. This stems from the fact that what you have already been thinking in your life is what has created the circumstances and situations of where you currently are. If you want something different, or more success than you have right now, then it means shifting your mindset and your thinking to more empowering thoughts.

Sharon Gorman, D.C.

When I first moved to Marietta, GA to become a chiropractor at Life Chiropractic College, I was only seventeen years old. I grew up in a middle-income family in a nice community where our household income was on the low side compared to our neighbors. Most of my friend's parents made more money than my parents and we attempted for it to not appear that way. At the time, I didn't have an abundant mindset. We "got by," never saving money and never donating to local charities or causes. When I arrived in Marietta, GA, I had no prior experience with a full-time job or awareness of financial abundance.

I started going to seminars where I'd vehemently watch the successful doctors. I observed their posture, how they saw themselves and appeared to others, how they dressed, and even how they tipped their waitresses. I decided to model myself after them and in doing so, my mindset began to change. I now saw myself

The 8 Laws of Chiropractic Success

as a successful chiropractor even as a teenager. I was never a starving student even though I lived on very little money. I was enjoying the process that would eventually take me where I wanted to go in chiropractic and in life. I figured if these other chiropractors could do it, so could I — and I did.

My goal was to be an ultra-successful chiropractor and person. I didn't have to wait until I was successful or became a chiropractor to start seeing myself that way. I just needed to start seeing it. The internal changes were happening quietly between my ears. I watched the winners and I saw myself as one of them. After graduation, It didn't take me very long in practice to manifest ultra-success because that was what I was already seeing in my mind's eye as a student. I created a different mindset, not waiting around for it to happen or for someone else to do it for me. This is what I recommend you do too.

People have always looked at me and said, "Well if she can do it so can I." Many of my associates, after leaving my employ, would say that one of my special qualities is that I make becoming successful and being successful look easier than what they've heard and experienced. That's because in my mind I am successful. I don't struggle to become successful or worry about being successful because I already am successful. It all comes from my mindset — SEEING MYSELF — as a successful chiropractor, which became anchored within me so many years ago.

Larry Markson, D.C.

You must have an "inside-out" rather than an "outside-in" perspective or else you cannot possibly realize your fullest practice and life potential. Your view must be unlimited. After all, your outer life always mirrors your inner self, not the other way around.

Eighty percent of the world is in a loop, like an old cassette tape. They think if they DO this, they will HAVE that ... and if they HAVE this, they will BE that. They live in a world of "Do, Have, Be."

The other 20 percent adopt the more useful approach of

"Be, Do, Have." They know that who they are determines what they get: the way they think, walk and stand; the people they hang out with; the books they read; the television programs they watch; the environment they create; and the friends they make.

It's the limited "stinkin' thinkin'" that comes from parents, teachers, and preachers in the past that keeps you from developing a new mindset.

Lou Corleto, D.C.

If you have a "treatment consciousness," it's going to be really challenging for you because you are treating conditions and symptoms, which are only teaching tools used by the Innate Intelligence in the body. You're playing with a superficial experience — which can potentially drive you nuts.

You must see that a person's symptoms and conditions are not something meant to be attacked and gotten rid of. Instead, you need to view them as helpful messages from another level, as communication to the individual and the practitioner. There has to be a willingness on the part of the practitioner to see things differently.

Practitioners who have a mindset of service should remember something that Donny Epstein, D.C., so eloquently said, "Take no credit, take no blame." That doesn't mean becoming apathetic. Rather, it means you must always improve and master your ability to articulate the chiropractic message through education and empowerment, as well as deliver the goods through the adjusting process. As long as you are doing that, then "Take no credit, take no blame."

Tedd Koren, D.C.

You must have a sense of purpose and a calling to do this work. This is not about disease treatment and the practice of medicine. It is something that has incredible potential. Years ago, many of those who went to chiropractic school were themselves cured of horrible diseases and were living testimonials.

Today, you find that many of the students going to chiropractic college have never been adjusted. They come into it thinking that it's a good profession where they'll make lots of money and be secure. There's nothing wrong with any of that stuff but there's quite a bit more to it than that, wouldn't you say?

Paul Reed, D.C.

Mindset is a key ingredient in the reception of life. Unfortunately, many of us accept the place of victim to our circumstances and mediocrity by allowing external influences of parents, friends, coaches, and the like to affect our belief patterns. If you can master listening to your innate voice of abundance you'll break the chains of disbelief and doubt.

There are multiple training methods out there to help with programing your mindset with unlimited potential. Applying some of these simple tools to your daily rituals will help with hitting the daily reset button, allowing a clean slate towards growth and success.

You've seen it time and time again, those who overcome extreme obstacles, defy the odds, or survive near death experiences, learn to use the power of their mind to carry them through tumultuous times. Learning to tap into the power of your mindset may just be the difference between success and failure. Victory doesn't always go to the most talented warrior. It goes to the warrior who believes they can. So believe in yourself, your healing abilities, and that you are worthy of a fruitfully abundant life.

Kevin Jackson and Selina Sigafoose-Jackson, D.C.'s

As chiropractors we really take the idea seriously that mindset directly effects our practice. As we learned from the great James Sigafoose, D.C., our practice is a direct reflection of our mindset.

We spend the morning either reading spiritual messages and or meditating before entering the office.

Dick Santos, D.C., used to say, "You need to be like clean hollow bone so the spirit can work through you." Having a mindset that's devoid of fear, anger, jealousy, lust or greed is a great way to start your day in the chiropractic office. Unfortunately, Facebook doesn't prepare us to properly serve people in a chiropractic setting. So devoting time developing the proper mindset is essential for successfully serving chiropractic.

Teri and Stu Warner, D.C.'s

Your success in practice and in life depends entirely on one thing: your mindset. Do you have the winning mindset that will ensure your success?

We all have a mindset, an established set of attitudes or beliefs. They dictate how we live our lives, how we practice, and how we serve our patients. They will help establish your income, how fast your practice grows, and how you divide your time both personally and professionally.

When lecturing, we often ask chiropractors to share stories about their most memorable pediatric patients. As they present the story and share the miracle, their mindset is palpable. You can feel the intensity with which they cared for this child and how invested this doctor was in the outcome. This is the mindset of a winner, one who operates at the level of intensity necessary to tap into and reach the highest levels of success.

This mindset will influence your beliefs, your procedures, your adjusting skills, your management, your marketing success, and even your personality. Are these qualities "set in stone?" No. You have the opportunity to make tomorrow anything you want it to be. You can achieve this through love of success and dedication to changing the world.

For us, our mindset is to see every parent educated and every child receive the amazing benefits of chiropractic care from womb to tomb to maximize their health and wellbeing. Choose your own motivation, and if positive goal setting is somehow not enough for you, fear is usually a powerful motivator. Fear of failure, fear of your checks bouncing, and fear of living in a world full of subluxated individuals.

Don't be a wantrapreneur! Have the mindset and take the action steps to make your dreams a reality. Be bold, be powerful, be fearless, be committed, and be passionate! When you have the mindset of a champion, success is sure to follow.

Chapter 2

"Dreams are extremely important. You can't do it unless you can imagine it." - George Lucas

Law Two – Vision

David K. Scheiner, D.C.

What is it that you truly want? What do you desire and what makes you itch? What is it, if money were no object, would have you leap out of bed in the morning, and like my friend John Demartini says, "Where your vocation becomes your vacation so you tap dance to work every day?" Whatever that is, go do it and forget the money because when you truly love what you do the money is sure to follow. Are you practicing a certain way other than that which you hold dear to your own heart? Is there an incongruency within you with regards to your practice, relationships, or another area in your life? If there is then your vision is clouded.

Napoleon Hill said, "Whatever the mind can conceive and believe, the mind can achieve," and you know what, he's right. You must have a clear vision if you are to achieve anything great in life. Whatever it is, you must first be able to see it in your mind having already happened and then you go to work — backwards — merely filling in the pieces. It's like this book you're reading. I saw it finished and completed in my mind first, over a decade ago. I knew exactly who I was going to ask to be in it, what the title was, what the cover looked like, and the dimensions. I knew who was going to accept the invite to be in the book, who wasn't, and then I went to work filling in the pages to get it done. And Voilá, here it is!

It's the same way with your life. Know what it is you want and then see it having already happened in your vision. Then get to work filling in the blanks and work it backwards so you create and manifest it. It takes a large clear vision in your minds eye in order to light the path you'll follow to your magnificently manifested destination. Whatever you think about, positive or negative, you become. Whatever drives you, whatever those thoughts are on a constant basis, shapes your reality and present place in life.

Steve Jobs did this when creating Apple. He saw products in his vision first and then he and his team worked backwards, filling in the blanks, until their creation. He was a very spiritual man who was lit afire at a young age. One of the things that set him on the path was the book **Autobiography of a Yogi** by Paramahansa Yogananda. Jobs read that book many times throughout his life. At his funeral, each person was given a small brown box. In that box contained a copy of this book; that's how much of an impact it made on him. What books do that for you? What are you filling up your subconscious mind with that is creating your reality? Look into reading books on The New Thought Movement, The Science of Getting Rich by Wallace Wattles, As A Man Thinketh by James Allen, as well as The Game of Life and How To Play it by Florence Scovel Shinn.

What has you lit up? What is something new that you will create? If you are following in someone else's footsteps, muster up the courage to step to the right or left and create a new path for yourself. Infuse your life with a greater sense of mystery and newness by lessening the need to control. Don't allow yourself to be stuck inside a jail cell or box. Your job is to unlock peoples potentiality from within — not to be subluxated in your own mind. Without having the courage to create your new vision (future) you will get more of your past. The world needs what your vision projects onto it; allow yourself space to create freely so that your vision for humanity touches, moves, and inspires the masses.

The 8 Laws of Chiropractic Success

Chuck Ribley, D.C.

My mindset is the platform for my vision, my dream. Quoting B.J. Palmer, D.C., from **The Bigness of the Fellow Within** — chapter one That Something, "The most important thing one can do is to awaken to that something within and let it become the guiding force in your life."

From this inspiration within comes to ALL people the books, the songs, and the inspiration, etc. of your reason to BE! I had my walking papers when I graduated from Palmer College in 1960. Go out into the world and adjust the 7 billion people, then come back and you will receive your next order.

Tim Young, D.C.

To have vision is one of the key cornerstones of chiropractic success. Some mistake vision as being able to see in their mind where they want to go. I believe the vision that is most required for success is the ability to see where you currently are. The present time conciseness, being aware of who you are at each given moment is the secret. Your focused moments turn into hours, days, months, and eventually when the years start adding up you realize your vision.

Kevin Jackson and Selina Sigafoose-Jackson, D.C.'s

The vision we've always had is to serve as many people as possible for the sake of humanity and not for the sake of ourselves. Of course we understand how elementary it is to first take care of ourselves so that we may serve others. But a sustained vision of helping humanity has given us strength in the long run.

We have been at an extremely high level of practice for 30 years and have never become bored or burned out. The vision of bringing chiropractic to the world helps us keep working Friday afternoon and Saturday mornings. The vision of helping thousands of people per month live a life free of nerve interference is really quite invigorating.

The 8 Laws of Chiropractic Success

At this point in time almost 20,000 people have come through our doors that we've imparted the chiropractic vision on. Whether they've rejected or accepted the ideas, we believe we're doing our part to move the chiropractic lifestyle forward.

Jim Dubel, D.C.

I see myself, and every other Chiropractor, as a healer. Having been given the gift and knowledge of Chiropractic, we are the ones who can, will, and must change the world. Imagine every child being checked and adjusted from the moment of birth, what an incredible difference that would make in the world.

Imagine if every person in one city was adjusted, how that city would change. Imagine if every person in that state was adjusted, how that state would change. What if every person in the country was adjusted? How would the country change? Now, imagine if every person in the WORLD was adjusted, how that would change the entire world for the better! This is my vision for myself, for you, and for the world.

Jeanne Ohm, D.C.

I remember a long time ago somebody said that if you want your community to come to you, you have to see beyond your community and have a vision of yourself reaching a larger group. If you want to see beyond your community, you have to see your state, then your country, and ultimately the entire world. You have to realize that this is a global thing and the effect you have goes beyond the individuals who come into your office.

According to the new sciences, every time you affect one aspect of life, you are affecting all aspects of life. Expand your vision. It's so much bigger than how many people you see a week, how many people you have under a care plan, or whatever those small things are that consume you day to day. If you focus only on those figures, you'll always feel guilty that you didn't see enough patients or didn't meet your numbers. In that realm, you're trying to control and regulate a flow. That is not what this is all about.

Billy DeMoss, D.C.

Vision ties into purpose and drive. Being a visionary requires engaging with the creative aspects of your imagination while planning out where you're going to lead our profession and planet. Getting everyone in the world to understand what true chiropractic is about should be your primary vision. So many people have pigeonholed chiropractic but the picture is so much bigger and brighter; ripe for you to take it to the masses.

Everyone has been exposed to, compromised, and suppressed by toxicity on a variety of levels. My goal is for humanity to be elevated passed the normal levels so they may express their creative side and actualize their own beautiful inner visions of themselves.

Vision is purpose and it's why you get up in the morning. Without a clear vision you have no direction, desire, or drive. You're like a ship without a compass, merely being taken to and fro, in the direction that the winds and ocean waves are pushing you. Set goals, write affirmations, and visualize your mission; most importantly, do the work to achieve it.

∞

Liam Schubel, D.C.

In my smash hit book CAST TO BE CHIROPRACTORS, I open with a quote, "The bigger the vision, the bigger the life." Having a big vision helps you to bring the focus of your efforts onto a goal that is bigger than just yourself. The bigness of your vision can define the level of action that is required from you on a daily basis. So many chiropractors and students live mediocre lives by their own design. They focus on just getting by rather than living for something much bigger than themselves. As a result they lack

The 8 Laws of Chiropractic Success

the drive to execute the actions that could catapult them to a higher expression of themselves.

The vision I have maintained in my mind's eye since being a student is the following, "A world where every man, woman, and child has the opportunity to be checked for vertebral subluxation and adjusted when necessary from birth. Every day one must ask oneself if their actions are in alignment with their values and vision. The very thot of your vision should move you to take more constant action! If your goals are also in alignment with that vision then you live in a state of accomplishment and gratitude as your begin to realize that your existence as a chiropractor is truly crucial to the transformation and evolution of the planet.

A successful vision based chiropractic business is one that has clearly defined systems. Each system is innovated and refined to meet the needs of the business while aligning with the vision. Every position in your organization is contracted to bring about the vision. Every player on your team understands that they too play a key role in bringing about a vision bigger than themselves. In essence, your business becomes a business worth operating. People in your business will have a greater level of job satisfaction, motivation, and energy because they understand their value in bringing about a vision greater than themselves.

John Demartini, D.C.

Any detail you leave out of your vision is an obstacle you'll face in your office. The vitality of your practice is going to be in direct proportion to the vividness of the vision. Any time you have unclear vision, you are going to have hesitancy and that will result in a leveling off of the progress in your office.

Many of my clients say their practice has plateaued and they don't seem to be able to attract more patients. I ask them what future they see for themselves and it's usually a vague cliché about success. They do not have any real clarity about what they are going to do and the actions required to get there.

The 8 Laws of Chiropractic Success

Vitality is built on vision, and if you have a clear vision, you'll automatically surround yourself with, and want to be around, people who also have clear vision. If you do, your practice grows automatically.

D.D. Humber, D.C.

"Without vision the people will perish." Believe it or not, I was first introduced to the concept of visualization as a student at Palmer School of Chiropractic in the early 1950's. I first thought the concept was rather strange, but I gradually came to realize just how important this concept was to one's ultimate success.

Meditation and visualization, when practiced on a regular basis, can open up one's subconscious mind to unlimited possibilities. To illustrate, when a baseball player is at bat, he must see the ball coming at him as big as a grapefruit. When he can do this, he will get more hits (by far) than a batter who sees the baseball coming at him the size of a golf ball. A player with this mindset while at the plate will struggle to attain a batting average of even .200!

∞

Teri and Stu Warner, D.C.'s

Rick Warren said, "My Imagination Influences My Aspiration." In other words, your dreams determine your destiny. To accomplish anything, you must first have a mission, a goal, a hope, and a vision.

As chiropractors, we need a clear and purposeful vision. However, if you understand and believe the fundamental principles and philosophy of chiropracTIC, the vision is easy to see and achieve.

We all need a vision for our lives, yet the sad reality is that many of your patients don't have a vision that inspires them. Worse yet, many have lost their purpose and enthusiasm for life and health. The good news is you have the opportunity to inspire, lead, and grow a tribe of health warriors in your practice and in your community!

The 8 Laws of Chiropractic Success

Years ago, one of the ways we honed our vision was to write our mission statement. With each word carefully chosen, we were able to define our goals for our life, our practice, our purpose and our vision. We knew we wanted to focus our practice on kids, but just saying that was too vague. We needed to define our avatar in specific detail.

The bottom line is that you get what you focus on and it can be easy to get lost in the noise and excitement of your life. Without a clear direction, you'll spin your wheels and never get anywhere. Start by focusing on and clarifying your vision by writing your mission statement, followed by specific goals with timelines and dates.

Ask yourself, "How many patients do I want to serve per day and per week? What percentage of kids and pregnant woman do I want to help?" Next, use your mission statement to create a vision board for your office and your life, making sure to include personal, self-development, spiritual growth, health, diet, body, fitness, and financial goals. This vision becomes a powerful, driving force, that once unleashed, will make your dream practice and life a reality! Now you have the unique opportunity to make your life a masterpiece, to live what you teach, and to walk your talk.

Tedd Koren, D.C.

It is all about one's vision. One of mine is to have a school someday. Philosophy is vision. What do you see? What are your goals? What is healing to you? The number one reason people become healers is to learn how to heal themselves. For thousands and thousands of years there has been an understanding of the "journey of the wounded healer." We become healers so we may have a better opportunity to heal ourselves and in learning to heal ourselves, we may then heal others.

Having patients is one of the best ways to learn how to heal yourself because you get all these great examples of people with challenges. Many of their challenges reflect those we see in ourselves. We can run away from them, stay in denial, and refuse to deal with our issues, or we can open up and deal with the pain (it's always painful to see where you're lacking, where you hurt) and then move on to heal it. I can assure you that it will involve pain; being uncomfortable is part of the healing process.

Janice Hughes, D.C.

I've been so fortunate to be around amazing coaches and mentors in my Chiropractic life; originally as a student, then in practice, and ultimately as a Chiropractic Coach and Leader. So many of these people had incredible visions and I can vividly remember many moments of questioning myself, "How I could ever be that crystal clear?" I 'got' that the clarity of my vision is what would draw me to attract all the right people and things to facilitate creating just that. Yet what was I to do when I didn't have the next five, ten, and twenty years clearly in my mind?

Then I discovered coaching and realized that clarity didn't have to be for a defined amount of time in years. Instead of feeling 'less than,' if I could just ask myself more empowering questions and focus on what I did see into the next stage of my future, then I could attract all the resources and opportunities to create that vision!

I recommend taking a piece of paper and a pen and write these questions down now:

- If there were no rules, and I couldn't fail, what would I love my life to look like?
- Where do I envision my practice in 12 – 18 months?
- What would happen in my business and life if I increased my profitability?
- Who do I need to be or become to build a world class Chiropractic Business?

Hidden within your answers to these questions, and your commitment to writing down your insights, is your Vision!

The 8 Laws of Chiropractic Success

Brad Glowaki, D.C.

"It's not the view, it's the vision" is a sign that hangs above my desk and it's something everyone in the chiropractic profession needs to understand. It should not be about where you are but where you want to be.

All too often chiropractors get wrapped up in what is immediately in front of them, failing to recognize, or what's worse, failing to *identify* their vision — limiting themselves in the process.

It is where you are looking that you generally will ascend to. Therefore, as a profession, it is key that we not only elevate our mindset, but also operate with a bigger vision in mind. For example, people can live healthier lifestyles and we can help them achieve that. We can save lives through the power of chiropractic. It is through this process that we will be able to move beyond the mere mechanistic; making a larger, longer-lasting, and more positive impact in the communities we serve.

We are the answer so many are searching for. It's time we align our vision to match that.

Frederick A. Schofield, D.C.

Proverbs 29:18 state, *"Where there is no vision the people perish."* You have to have a vision. Vision creates visionaries, one who sees the bigger picture. You DeSire to see the vision expanding in your Consciousness. The vision must be bigger than money, bigger than survival, bigger than the big house, and a nice car.

"He who is uncertain hesitates and he who hesitates is like a wave of the sea agitated and tossed by the wind" said James 1:6. You are going to be thrown off course, that's a given. But when you have direction and a compelling vision, you will sustain your course. If your vision is too small, it has no attraction. Think of your vision in 3D like Disney World. Thru thots and intentions, that vision will manifest into Reality.

A practice without a vision is like a ship seeking a harbor

The 8 Laws of Chiropractic Success

without any guidance from a beacon or lighthouse. You are completely at the mercy of the wind, the waves, and the elements. If you have a vision, it will guide you to safe harbor.

From your vision, you can then translate that into your mission, and then into your purpose. You must use the power of your creative imagination to create the vision - anchoring it into the sensory afferent pathways with your thots, feelings, and actions and with that, you will translate your vision into reality.

Take out a piece of paper and write down your vision. Our vision was quite simple:

> *To master Clinical Excellence in Our Chiropractic practice and to communicate that with our patients.*
> *To serve as many patients as divinely possible. To have no barriers to access Chiropractic in Practice.*

Be Still and Sow and SO IT IS!!!

Joe Strauss, D.C.

First, you have to determine what your vision is. Is your vision to make a lot of money? Is it to be successful and have a great reputation in your community? If your vision is to do everything you can to get your community to understand what chiropractic is, all the other things are going to fall into place. I've found that the more I fulfill the vision of everybody in my community understanding what I do, the more people come into my office. All of my other ideas are going to then come to fruition and I'll reach all my other goals.

Gilles LaMarche, D.C.

Vision directly relates to the success of chiropractors and chiropractic students. Focused vision is an ability to see what you want to be, what you want to achieve, and clearly understand why. Sunlight focused through a magnifying glass can start a fire; how-

The 8 Laws of Chiropractic Success

ever, the conditions must be just right. If the magnifying glass is held too far from the surface, the rays are diffused and won't generate enough heat to make fire. When you heat water to 100°C it begins to boil. If the temperature only reaches 99°C, the water does not boil.

Why are some people and organizations more innovative, more influential, and more successful than others? Why do some command greater loyalty from customers, peers, and employees?

People such as Martin Luther King Junior, Steve Jobs, and the Wright brothers might have little in common but they all started with a vision and they all started by understanding their why. Their natural ability to start with the "why" enabled them to inspire those around them and to achieve remarkable results.

In his book **Start with Why: How Great Leaders Inspire Everyone to Take Action**, Simon Sinek states, "All great leaders who have the greatest influence in the world think, act, and communicate in the exact same way, and it's the complete opposite of what everyone else does." He calls this powerful idea *The Golden Circle*, and it provides a framework upon which organizations can be built, movements can be led, and people can be inspired.

It all starts with "why" and it all starts with a clear vision. To achieve what you want to achieve, whether passing exams and graduating with your Doctor of Chiropractic degree or achieving the practice of your dreams, you must be willing to have a definite aim for your life and truly give it your all. How clear is your vision and how willing are you to do whatever it takes to achieve it?

Cathy Wendland-Colby, D.C.

Some of you have sight and no vision. You look at life with your eyes and think what you see is all you can be.

When Life University lost its accreditation, enrollment dropped and money was tight (that's putting it nicely — they had to ration toilet paper). From the outside looking in, the profession saw the writing on the wall. Life was doomed. The board knew that what they didn't need was someone to follow the old plans. They needed someone with vision. Dr. Guy Riekeman came in with a 2020 vision — they'd lost the majority of their students and didn't have money for toilet paper — yet he was talking about building a livable campus. Now that's vision!

Vision is being able to see with your eyes closed, knowing that you are so much more than you've ever seen, and that you are far more capable, more powerful, and can certainly have a much greater impact than you do right now.

Your vision has to be massive to overcome your excuses. When you create a bigger vision for your life, a better vision of yourself, and when you can see where you're going with your eyes closed and believe in yourself, you will transform and so will the lives you touch.

Patrick Gentempo, D.C.

Vision is the foundation that all human beings must have in order to create something that doesn't currently exist. If you say to yourself, "I want to have a practice," then you have to have a vision for it before you can create it. If you're in a practice and want to double it, you have to have a vision for that before you can create it. Vision is the first step toward turning something you want into reality.

Ross McDonald and Rebecca Vickery, D.C.'s

Everyone ends up somewhere in life. A few people end up somewhere on purpose and with clarity. Those are the people with vision; having a clearly defined path or dream. Having a clear vision serves no purpose without the courage to take action and follow through. Humanity is littered with great geniuses and visionaries who have lacked the courage to follow through on their vision. Where do you see yourself fitting in with the progress of humanity?

The 8 Laws of Chiropractic Success

Without a vision to guide their day-to-day decisions, leaders are trapped in the tyranny of the urgent and the minutiae of the immediate day to day necessities. If you aim for nothing you will hit the target every time. Your energy, your vitality, and your focus becomes sharper — the more clear you are on your vision. Be clear in great detail on what you want to achieve. Dream big and take action on your vision and that will bring you great success.

Sharon Gorman, D.C.

It's hard to get somewhere if you don't know where you are going. James Sigafoose, D.C., used to tell me that many chiropractors would consult with him for advice about their practice because they felt like they were burnt out. He said to me, "They are not burnt out they are bored out." If I don't have a vision or goals that I am shooting for, I don't feel challenged. I feel I'm standing still. I need to be excited about where I am going, even after thirty-four years in practice.

There were times in my life when I didn't want to create a vision because I wanted to listen to my Innate Voice and try to live out God's will for me. By creating goals I was afraid I would take away the spontaneity by trying to force my will and desires on the world. For me, that was just an excuse not to dream. By allowing my mind to visualize and daydream I'm able to create a vision of where I think I would like to be. I am always aware that I don't control life, including any of the other people and many of the circumstances, so I can let it flow even while having a vision.

Your vision will change but that's no excuse not to dream. I used to selfishly think that the other people in my world should act the way I wanted them to. I know now that much of my disappointments and frustrations came from that disillusioned mindset. That mindset didn't work for me so I'm changing it. I'm choosing to change me, and I realize that works. You may need to take a self-inventory and notice what needs to change about yourself.

The 8 Laws of Chiropractic Success

It isn't taking a step backward when we change our vision and our self. That is actually growth. We'll find that, often times, what happens in our life exceeded our initial vision. If everything happens exactly the way we think it should, our life probably will be boring. Allowing your vision to change, as you change your vision, will always give you hope.

Reggie Gold, D.C.

It always comes back to the same thing. If you don't have a vision about what chiropractic is, how can you be successful at chiropractic? Those who consider themselves successful are really those who are making money out of the practice of medicine. Adjustment of a spine by hand is the practice of medicine if the intent is to get sick people well and prevent well people from getting sick. Chiropractic is only chiropractic in its pure sense when it's done for no other reason than to rid the body of subluxation. *Then* it's pure chiropractic.

We put in the force, which we hope the body will accept and convert into an adjustment. That's a technical thing. Chiropractors who think they're making the adjustments would have to know where the bone belongs, which they can't possibly know. That's medical thinking. Medical thinking says that all human beings are virtually alike and that the spine is supposed to be in the middle. The spine is not supposed to be in the middle. The spine is supposed to be where the body needs it to be in order to protect the spinal cord and its branches. That may be different in every human being, as no two people are alike.

The lamina may be a little thicker on one side in one person or more curved in another. We can't possibly know what the spine is really like with regard to its shape and thus we can't know where it's supposed to be.

Medical practitioners and medically thinking chiropractors put the spine where they think it should be, just as medical doctors try to regulate the temperature to what they think it should

The 8 Laws of Chiropractic Success

be. True chiropractors know it's none of their business what the temperature should be ... or where the bones should be. Their job is to correct any subluxations and allow the body to work by itself. They're not here to raise or lower temperature, to raise or lower blood pressure, or to raise or lower cholesterol. All we want to do is allow the body the freedom to express itself. True chiropractic is much simpler than most chiropractors realize.

Paul Reed, D.C.

Your vision is your roadmap in life. If you can't first see where it is you want to go, then how are you going to get there? Establishing crystal clear images of each category of your life (practice, relationships, finances, etc.) will decrease the amount of resistance you face getting there. Creating a vision helps align your path with the universe so that it is working with you instead of against you.

One of my early mentors worked with me on vision nearly twenty-one years ago. He had me write out a super descriptive vision of what I wanted my practice to look like. Every detail went in this manuscript from the size of the space, the colors on the walls, the tables, the images on the walls, the type of people I wanted to care for, the amount of people I wanted to serve, the music, the smells, and so on. Within three short years of implementing this exercise, we had the exact practice we had visualized.

I encourage every chiropractor and student to establish a clear vison for your practice and life. This will set the course of success in motion towards your dreams.

Christopher Kent, D.C.

Vision inspires action but without the implementation of action, the vision itself is nothing but an elegant abstract thing.

Thom Gelardi, D.C.

Success starts with a vision of what you wish to actualize. In the 7 Habits of Highly Successful People, Stephen R. Covey writes that we should start with the end. Big visions, and their plans, are easier to actualize than small ones. Daniel Burnham (famed architect and urban planner, 1846-1912) wrote, "Make no little plans; they have no magic to stir men's blood, and probably will themselves not be realized. Make big plans; aim high in hope and work..."

The more detailed the vision, the more likely its actualization. A comprehensive vision includes your state of health, character, family, relationships, practice, and standing in your profession. A vision must be translated into a plan with measurable goals, implemented through strategies and tactics. Life is a journey rather than a destination and its satisfaction and joy lies in the direction and quality of that journey.

Arno Burnier, D.C.

Vision is paramount, essential, and crucial. When I was in practice, my vision of a family wellness practice carried the day.

Amanda and Jeremy Hess, D.C.'s

Without Vision, we become wandering vessels adrift in the sea of life, who make little impact on society and fail to leave a legacy for future generations. Vision, many times, starts with the singular and over time grows into including more and more people, eventually becoming nothing about ourselves and everything about the people we serve.

The lives of future generations are positively impacted and inevitably affected by our working tirelessly on our vision throughout life. Most people have trouble creating or seeing their vision and purpose early in life or have such a small vision that it is mainly about themselves. Nothing is wrong with that in

The 8 Laws of Chiropractic Success

the beginning, as the main goal is to simply get moving in the right direction, taking action steps to become the person you wish to be.

As you formalize who you are and mature, cultivating what your purpose is in life, you will start to see your vision grow beyond yourself. Similar to Maslow's Law of Hierarchy, you grow and mature in Life with each success, realizing that you are not living this life for yourself but for others. Your vision will, on many levels, take on growth of becoming more about others needs, how you can give back, making an impact in your family, your community, and generations to come.

Have your vision expand exponentially like the ripples in a pond when a rock is thrown in. Go after your vision and don't be swayed by what others say to you or about you. Do not be dismayed. Follow your vision and don't look back or take heed in others opinions. Remember the words of B.J. Palmer, D.C., "Many people have the eyesight of a hawk, but the Vision of a clam."

Jessica Harden, D.C.

There is something to be observed and learned from people who don't focus and work towards a specific idea or purpose. These people can wander aimlessly through life, feeling bored, frustrated, or dissatisfied. Vision is not the same as a dream or wish. It is not superficial. Creating a vision is not as simple as waking up with an idea and suddenly deciding to work toward it. An idea can spark the vision, but that alone will not create it.

A vision requires self-reflection and time to create a very specific idea of who you are and what you desire to create in this world. The more specific your vision the easier it will be to know what you are willing to do—and what you are not willing to do. This clarity can transform your journey to success, making it easier to prioritize your time, saying no to distractions, and providing an anchor through difficult seasons.

Visions need time for development. To explore and create a

The 8 Laws of Chiropractic Success

specific vision, set aside time to disconnect, ponder on what brings you joy in life, and what that looks like for you. Don't be afraid to think big or far ahead. I once heard it said, "If you shoot for the stars, you will get the moon." Think of the impact your creation will make and most importantly write your thoughts down and constantly review. Consistently developing the clarity of your vision will guide your steps on the road to success.

Daniel & Richelle Knowles, D.C.'s

In the movie Butch Cassidy and the Sundance Kid, Butch says, "I'm a man of vision, and the whole world is wearing bifocals." Butch sees the world differently and in the movie he repeats that quote over and over.

Chiropractors and chiropractic students have a different vision of the world. Once you become a chiropracTOR, you have a pair of chiropracTIC goggles installed. They filter your vision where the world is seen through completely different eyes. It's as though you're living in a world where *you* know it's round and the *other* people see it flat. You've come to know the truth while *they* continue to exist within a completely different reality.

You now have an incredible gift to see Life as Life truly is. That TIC vision can be extremely far reaching and for some can even be blinding. When you truly get the BIG idea of chiropracTIC, you'll realize that it's the biggest idea you'll ever come to know. It will incorporate your biggest vision and encompass everything that you could ever imagine.

When I was a chiropractic student I went on a road trip with a bunch of fellow students. My chiropractic goggles had already been installed and while traveling, I saw a billboard on the side of the road, which amazingly read, *"There's magic in a healthy spine."* I was completely astounded and impressed that a chiropractor put up a billboard focusing on the positive outcomes when one has a healthy spine, instead of putting the danger signs of neck pain, back pain, headaches, or symptoms.

The 8 Laws of Chiropractic Success

Unfortunately, no one else in the car at the time saw that sign but me. I told everyone on the trip about it and couldn't wait to point it out upon our return. As we approached the sign

There's magic in a healthy spine!

I excitedly said to them, "Look, there it is up ahead!" As we slowly approached, we all laughed realizing that, instead of it reading *"There's Magic In A Healthy Spine,"* it said *"There's Magic In A Healthy Smile."* It was a sign for a dental office!

Everything you see is impacted by your vision. When discussing the bigness of chiropractic with your practice members, realize that they do not have those same goggles installed in their eyes like you do and therefore it requires you to bring them along slowly and at their own unique pace. Chiropractic incorporates the biggest idea on the planet and as such requires people like you who have the biggest visions.

Gerard Clum, D.C.

As Sid Williams, D.C. used to say, "It's tough to remember that your job is to drain the swamp when you are up to your ass in alligators."

If your vision is of unemployment, failing banks, dropping property values, etc., that's not a positive vision. But, if your vision encompasses the long haul of the system, the cyclical nature of things, and the concept of cause and effect, then you recognize that the current situation is a reasonably predictable moment, and we'll move through it.

Vision gives you the ability to see over the long-term and perceive connections that other people don't see. One of the things I've been very fortunate to have is a sense of how things connect, an ability to see relationships that other people often don't notice. It looks clairvoyant at times but it's really just a matter of looking at the roadway from a different vantage point.

∞

Jason Deitch, D.C.

Your vision is the picture you create for your life and your practice. Do you have a vision that comes from within? Do you have a vision of a practice and communication style you want to model after? The vision you see in your mind is what drives your investment of effort, time, and money to achieve. Your vision is the dream you choose to create and the possibilities you choose to believe are possible.

So what's your dream? What contribution do you want to make in the world? Decades from now, when you look back on your life, what do you want to reflect on and see that you did with your days, weeks, months, and years? What type of practice do you want to build? What type of people do you want to serve? What type of business model do you want to operate? What type of service do you want to provide? Go ahead and take a piece of paper and pen out now and write those questions down. Spend some time answering them. Don't leave your life and practice to chance. What will you look back on and be most proud of?

The answers to these above questions are the blue print of your success. They drive the actions you take and the life you build for yourself. So choose wisely, dream big, and most importantly, dream often.

Larry Markson, D.C.

Vision is huge. People often say that someone is visionary simply because that person is successful but a real visionary can look into the future. Lee Iacocca could see seven years into the future and there were others who could see further than that.

Every single person has to have a vision, a mission statement, and a purpose greater than the everyday, tangible, physical world. In chiropractic, a goal might be to adjust one-hundred people a day or three hundred to five hundred people a week. But that's not a mission statement. A mission statement is, "To help as many people as possible." There is a vision!

The 8 Laws of Chiropractic Success

My vision is to create an environment where I can help as many people as I can get well naturally without taking anything from outside and putting it inside the body so that the human body can express its potential. That is a vision. It's greater than the notion of just banging a spine so the person feels better.

Guy Riekeman, D.C.

Vision creates involvement. Patients whose vision of health care is simply getting from the antalgic position with a hot low back to standing up straight and be able to swing a golf club are going to be gone after seven visits. That's their level of involvement. If you can't change their vision of chiropractic while they are there, then their level of involvement is always going to be the same.

Vision is the most critical factor to change involvement of a patient in a practice, of a chiropractor in a profession, and a student in college. Vision is about involvement.

Terry A. Rondberg, D.C.

Vision is where the intention comes from. If you have a vision then you can have an intention to reach it or to at least strive to reach it. Living or practicing without first creating a vision is like getting in your car and driving without knowing where you want to go. You may end up in some interesting places and may even enjoy the trip, but you might also wind up driving in circles and getting nowhere. If you have a clear destination in mind and map out your route, you can be almost sure to arrive at your goal. That doesn't mean the road trip is any less enjoyable, but at least you aren't going to be stuck in Podunk when you really want to be in Boston!

Applying that analogy to chiropractic is simple. If you get to your office each day without having a true, clear vision of what you want your practice to be, you're going to go around in circles. If you're real lucky, you may end up having a successful practice but do you really want to depend on dumb luck?

The 8 Laws of Chiropractic Success

Instead, spend some time to pick your destination with care. Think about what you REALLY want out of your practice, not just about the income you hope to achieve. Would it make you happier and more fulfilled to work three days a week pro bono at homeless shelters? If yes, create a vision of yourself doing that, and fill in all the details of that vision. See yourself giving adjustments to those who would never otherwise be able to receive the gift of chiropractic. Feel the sense of satisfaction that comes with service.

Understand, too, that there's no "right or wrong" when it comes to your vision. No one has any business judging the relative merits of what you want for yourself and your practice. Even if some people do make judgments, you don't have to pay attention to them. It's your life and you deserve to live it the way you choose!

CJ Mertz, D.C.

The practice we see in the future is perfect; the one we have right now is imperfect. You need to visualize the practice you want to have. Who is your ideal patient? What's your ideal day? What kind of person is your ideal CA? What's your ideal practice? As you think, ponder, contemplate, and meditate on that vision, you are actually creating the perfection of that practice environment in the future.

Of course, there are no mistakes in your vision. Your vision is perfect. While your practice of today is full of mistakes and imperfections, the one you see in the future is flawless.

Put a little bit of perfection into our present imperfection...

The key is to be able to go into your vision and see what is perfect and then inject it into the present. Go forward into the future, see it perfect, and bring a little of that perfection back into today's imperfection. That's the foundation for constant and never-ending improvement: put a little bit of perfection into our present imperfection as we move forward. We can't do that without studying our vision on a daily basis.

The 8 Laws of Chiropractic Success

Brian Kelly, D.C.

Vision is the ideal state you wish to see in the future. If your vision for a person who presents in your practice with acute Low Back Pain and radiculopathy is to *only* get them out of pain and back to work or avoid surgery, this may be the highest vision you have for them.

It's not a right or wrong issue, it is a question of how big the ideal state you imagine for your patients is. Conversely, if your vision for the same patient is seeing them with a healthy spine and nerve system, and you are concepting the health and full genetic expression of their (yet) unborn grandchildren, you have created a greater vision of possibility for them.

Is the vision of your life as a chiropractor to only be comfortable and make a nice living or is your vision to change the world? Your answer to this will lead you towards one of two very different lives.

∞

Armand Rossi, D.C.

If you don't have a vision of where you want to go, you're aimless. You have to have a mission, a purpose, and a goal. It's really best to write them down so they enter the physical universe. Even if you don't write them down, you have to work to maintain that vision of where you want to go. Your vision gives you a focus point.

∞

Claudia Anrig, D.C.

Vision is the concept you capture in your mind that drives you to move forward into the future. When you have the vision of something, you know it three dimensionally and it becomes part of your life. Everybody's vision is different and that's what makes us unique from each other.

Capturing that vision propels you forward. If your vision is to begin and end a race, you see the finish line and that's where you'll go. The funny thing is, by the time you get to the finish line, you'll have captured a new vision to go even further. It's all about capturing something in your mind that you're going to work towards.

Lou Corleto, D.C.

Those with a sense of vision can start bringing future ideals to the here and now so you can actualize the original tenet of chiropractic, which is to help humanity make transitions. We play a vital role, through our vision, in making people's growth and spiritual transitions easier, more efficient, and gentler.

When I initially saw and understood the concept of transition and its relation to helping humanity, it hit home for me in many respects. Let's say you're serving moms and babies in the birthing process — you're helping the infants transition from one world to this one. Serving people who are taking their last breath is helping them make a transition from this world to the next.

When we serve people, we help them consciously make transitions from one state of consciousness to the next. Wherever they are in their growth phase — in and out of this world, in their own mental dynamics or emotional bodies — the adjusting process allows them to make that transition with much more grace and peace.

∞

Neil Cohen, D.C.

Vision is a valued and acquired gift that requires great courage combined with a deep and unshakable faith to make things happen. Ultimately it is creating your future. One who is a true visionary can see the existence and reality of things that have not yet begun to take place. They are virtually seeing an idea (in the future) in full fruition even before a strategy is applied. To have vision is to declare the end right from the beginning.

To think and speak in generalities is the antithesis of vision. Specificity is the core of vision and for the chiropractor and chiropractic student, it starts with a simple yet profound question, "What do I want?"

The 8 Laws of Chiropractic Success

Responding to this seemingly basic question, the chiropractor that has only sight but lacks the necessary vision may very well say, "I want to see more new patients" or "I want to have the most successful practice in my community."

The vision deprived student will say, "I'm going to be a doctor someday and I'm going to make lots and lots of money."

In each of these scenarios, which are comprised of mere hopeful notions, both the chiropractor and the student are lacking the required specificity for true vision. These declarative sentences are an imagined wish-list to be given over to hope, forever lacking the certainty needed for the desired outcome.

All visionaries know that deep desire alone is not enough. They are keenly aware that specificity is what crystallizes any vision, making the manifestation of it even more certain. As for the chiropractic warrior, whether student or licensed D.C., this specific "made up mindset" is the subtle difference between ones success or a future mired in mediocrity.

Steve Judson, D.C.

Without vision the people perish. Plain and simple. Just look at the world around you. It's as though we live in a vision-less society; where it's up to the chiropractic profession to provide people with their true sight. Through your minds-eye you must create a vision beyond what your current eyes will allow you to see.

Your spirit is unseen yet sees so much more than your inherent vision allows. You must paint a crystal clear outcome of what you want your life to look like and then build that vision brick by brick. You must see it every day and know where the next brick will go before you lay it down.

Dr. Sid taught us meditation and breathwork at Dynamic Essentials Seminars for a reason. He knew that this sacred space is where you create, build, and actualize your vision. See it and develop it everyday, while understanding that it is beyond reality where greatness sleeps. You must just see it and create the picture

The 8 Laws of Chiropractic Success

you want in order to actualize your vision. This takes work and it is not easy. What's the alternative?

Donny Epstein, D.C.

What are the highest short and long term impacts you envision when you interact with your practice member? The term practice member is one that I "coined" in 1982 to refer to an individual seeking care in a collaborative way where chiropractic is a strategy towards creating a higher order participatory perspective on healing and life.

Your vision must transcend the quest for comfort or restoring your practice member to a prior state. Instead, focus towards helping individuals to reorganize their personal energetic resources for a higher order existence, going beyond their ordinary level of health or healing.

Your vision and results are proportionate to how large you consider the system that you and your practice members participate in. Is the system you seek to impact consist of: the vertebrae, the subluxation, the inter-relations between the parts, the innate intelligence, the person's interactions in the field, their beingness, their coherence locally or globally, how they interact with others, and their health physically, emotionally, mentally, and spiritually?

Does your vision consider the unique aspects of the individual or the environment, and how their greater coherence impacts the field around them more than the environment impacting and downsizing the individual? Does your vision include specific outcomes? Simply said, the larger the system you envision, the larger your impact will be.

Chapter 3

"Our intention creates our reality." – Wayne Dyer

Law Three – Intention

David K. Scheiner, D.C.

Many years ago I watched the movie Don Juan DeMarco starring Johnny Depp, Marlon Brando, and Faye Dunaway. I recommend you watch it as soon as possible if you have not already seen it. There is a memorable line in the movie when Don Juan (Depp) says, "There are only four questions of value in life, Don Octavio (Brando). What is sacred? Of what is the spirit made? What is worth living for, and what is worth dying for? The answer to each is the same: only love." When we think about intention, when we do anything in life, whether it be work, family, personal, or wellness related we must intend to do it only with love. Love is the common denominator; the spark that makes the entire universe come alive.

In fact, if we are in something for any other reason, we must either transform our relatedness with it or gently remove ourselves from that equation or else we will be in for much turmoil, unhappiness, and despair. Intention comes first and then action, which is Law 8 (and the Law of Infinity). Ask yourself right now these questions and make some notes to your answers:

What's my intention with this life?
What did I come here to accomplish?
What do I hold most sacred to my heart?

If I am not living the life I imagined, what shift must I make to get on that track NOW?

When you feel scattered and unfocused, your intention becomes clouded. In life there are times that we get off track and slip. It is at these times that you ought to practice the art of grounding and centering yourself. Meditate holding specific crystals in each hand; hold them with the intention of balancing and cleansing each chakra. Picture all of the colors and then, one at a time, open each chakra and then close it when that level is complete. You'll be pulled back into balance, have brought color and resonance in, you will experience no more exhaustion, and your intentions will be pure once again.

Work with shifting what you do by intentionally stopping and starting it; think and do a little differently in order to add contrast to your life. Slowly add the richness of your soul and spirit into whatever you are doing and intend to become what you came here to be. Ask the question, "Who am I and what do I intend to bring to the world?" Upon the answer to that question rests your entire life.

Guy Riekeman, D.C.

The concept of intention can be better understood through the science of quantum physics. We know there's a field of possibility that has no space or time and it's from this field that we create the physical reality we live in.

On the level of subatomic particles, if you look in one direction, they show up there. But if you look in the other direction, they're no longer where they were; they're now where you are looking. There's a point where you move from this realm of possibility into the realm of physical reality at that moment. Intention is what creates that realm of transformation.

One scientific view of the beginning of the universe (and you can read Nobel Laureate and physicist Leon Lederman's book "The God Particle" to learn more) is that a supersaturated field of possibility existed with no space, time, or energy. Into that field of possibility came the energy of a thought. Since there was no place for it to go, the energy of the thought exploded into a massive amount of energy and some of these waves of energy began to synchronize and create the physical universe that we see.

The question has always been, "Where did that thought come from?"

The question for scientists has always been, "Where did that thought come from?" Einstein concluded that there must be a God. A lot of scientists believe that it came from a place called Higgs Field. There are all sorts of arguments surrounding this theory but ultimately it's about intention. An intent came into this field of possibility and from that intent the entire physical universe was formed.

We know that happens — just read Dr. Joe Dispenza's books or watch the movie "What the Bleep Do We Know?" It's all about creating the physical world we live in by creating intention. If your intention is to create a successful practice you will. If your intention is to create health you will.

Brad Glowaki, D.C.

If your intention is to take people out of pain, while achievable, that is ultimately the level of impact you are going to have. However, if your intention is to literally save lives year after year, then you will have a higher level of impact on the lives of those you serve in your communities.

Practicing with this higher level of intention, you are going to provide your patients with the opportunity to use the power of chiropractic to be the catalyst for the change they wish to see in their lives.

Ultimately, if your intentions are at a higher vibration, and independent of selfish means, then you are ultimately going to see a higher level of health in your community as a result.

The 8 Laws of Chiropractic Success

Janice Hughes, D.C.

Intent + Action = Magic

Most of us live our lives of daily 'to do' lists and checklists of actions. Yet why can I give this same list of actions to ten people and almost all of them get different results? I believe it's because of who they are, who they BE, and the intentions they bring to that list.

Even spending a few minutes per day focused on intention shifts your reality.

Intention doesn't always mean conscious thoughts — it is generally found in the silence. By listening to the 'whispers in the wind' you tap into intuition and inner guidance. Intention lives at the level of intuition.

Gilles LaMarche, D.C.

The Oxford dictionary defines intention as, "A thing intended; an aim or plan, the healing process of a wound, conceptions formed by directing the mind towards an object," but intention to me is even more than that. Intention is focus so clear that you see nothing else in that moment other than what you are intending to create.

> **You get what you intend to create by being in harmony with the power of intention...**

Carlos Castaneda said, "In the universe there is an immeasurable, indescribable force which shamans call intent and absolutely everything that exists in the entire cosmos is attached to intent by a connecting link."

My dear friend and mentor Dr. Wayne Dyer said, "If you aren't doing what you love and loving what you do, your **power of intention** is weakened. You attract into your life more of the dissatisfaction that isn't the face of love .... You get what you intend to create by being in harmony with the power of intention, which is responsible for all of creation."

The 8 Laws of Chiropractic Success

Dr. Larry Markson taught me a powerful lesson many years ago — to connect with intention with each patient / practice member before entering a room. At eye level on the outside door frame of every room, I stuck a small round purple sticker. I would briefly review their chart, internally connect with the person I was about to see, set the intention for the visit, and when ready I'd say to myself, "Guide me to do what is right for this person today." Once I experienced that connection, I would touch the purple dot, knowing that I was focused on that person, and ready to serve with focused intention.

Frederick A. Schofield, D.C.

Well the question is, "What is your intention?" If your intention is to be successful, then you would say: *"I intend to be successful in practice now."* Thots and intentions create your reality. Thots are things. Again thots and intentions create your reality!

Affirm:

"I intend to … create a successful practice now!"

Massive intentions create massive action.

We have two minds: we have the iNNATE mind (wisdom, love, compassion — the hippocampus) and then we have the dysfunctional mind (fear, anger — the amygdala). We have an intention in chiropractic to adjust our minds to alignment creating, *"When in alignment, the power that made the body heals the body."*

The healing power is accessed through the adjustment. We activate the iNNATE Divine Design in the organism thru the adjustment. The adjustment of the alignment thru our thots and intentions multiplied by space, time, and repetition creates the intention to be healthy.

1) Get Clear on your DeSires
2) You do not have to know how it is going to happen
3) Get it down on paper and Affirm: *"My thots and my intentions create my reality"*

The 8 Laws of Chiropractic Success

"I intend to attract Double Digit new patients per week and it shall be done unto me as I have faith."

Thots and intentions create your reality.

Be Still and Sow and SO IT IS!!!

Teri and Stu Warner, D.C.'s

Living and practicing with intention, rather than by chance, is paramount to personal and professional success. Having the mindset or will to concentrate on a goal, with a specific end or purpose in mind, is the difference between success and failure. Our intention becomes a spotlight, continuously demonstrating whether or not we're on the right path.

Let's take a look at a simple yet powerful example of intention in action. Go through your inactive patient list and put your intention on those patients who you haven't seen in some time. Within the next day or two, several of those patients will walk through your door without you or they ever making a phone call, sending a text, email, etc. for an appointment — the intention alone was enough.

It is your intention that determines the direction, flow, volume, income, and ultimate success (whatever that means to you) of your practice. You first see the vision in your mind's eye and then it may come to fruition. I see myself adjusting five-hundred people per week, I see my office filled with children, pregnant women, and babies. I see my bank account overflowing with revenue, I see chronic and difficult cases walking through my door, and I see a line of cars waiting to enter my parking lot.

It is equally important to have the proper intention behind your adjustment by focusing on the outcomes you desire. If your intention for the adjustment is to remove nerve interference, therefore allowing the body to thrive, have that be your focus.

Start your week off right by setting your intentions and asking yourself these questions: "What will I accomplish this week? How will I make this week better than the last? What is the one step I will take this week to grow my practice? How will I learn to focus my intention while delivering each and every adjustment with precision and skill? How much am I missing out on each day, each month, or each year by not focusing my intention? and How much increase can I see in my life immediately if I'd only switch my intent?"

With focused intention you can see more patients and facilitate more health and healing than you've ever thought possible. Your vision and ability to impact the world by impacting your community can remain local or go global, it is as boundless as your mindset. Expand your vision and expand your practice!

Cathy Wendland-Colby, D.C.

Have you ever heard the saying, "It's not the gift you give, it's the thought that counts?" Try telling that to a five-year-old who just opened a box full of clothes on Christmas morning. When you shopped, were you thinking of the desires of the recipient or of a need you had to fill? Maybe the child needed more clothes, or you needed less time spent on laundry, or you wanted them to look cute or make you look significant in the eyes of others. Why you do something can often overshadow what you do.

Why do you seek out new patients? Are you trying to fill your own need for money, status, or bragging rights to your colleagues? Or do you genuinely care about educating and empowering your community to raise healthy and unmedicated families?

When you are with a patient, is your intention to detect and correct vertebral subluxations, removing interference to the transmission of mental impulses, allowing for the restoration and maintenance of health? Or are you chatting away about meaningless minutia while thumping on their backs to make them feel better?

As you care for the newborns, speak into their subconscious about your intention, "Baby, right now I'm checking your spine

The 8 Laws of Chiropractic Success

for any misalignments which could interfere with your brain's ability to communicate with the rest of your body and as we remove the interference, every cell in your body will begin to function at a higher capacity, allowing you to grow and express your fullest human potential."

Billy DeMoss, D.C.

Intention is what you want to bring to fruition — it's what creates your purpose and drive. Say your intention is to make a lot of money. That's not something that's going to drive a meaningful purpose because money is just a vehicle and not an end. As Brad Glowaki says, "It should be the fine shavings of a fine carpenter."

My intention is to bring chiropractic to the world and make it known and available to everyone from the day they're born until their final breath. I want the world to know that chiropractic is not a pain-based model. My intention is to educate chiropractors, chiropractic students, and the world about a different paradigm, one of vitalism, steering everyone away from the medical mindset. Intention is vital and what you want to bring into the world.

Steve Judson, D.C.

Intention is everything and Dr. Sid always taught us that we must lose ourselves in service. When your vision is focused on serving others, true abundance is achieved. An intention of pure gain will only darken your vision. However, when your service to mankind is through love, this is an intention that will literally move mountains and bring a smile upon the entire universe.

When your heart is clear and connected to the source, it works through you at levels you could never have imagine before. Pure intention yields pure results each and every time. You must love first and then all else follows.

Paul Reed, D.C.

Intention is a powerful tool. The more focused your intention the faster you will create your life's vision. Having specific intentions will move you towards your goals, dreams, desires, and have you come across to people in an authentic and genuine manner.

I once had a CrossFit coach tell me, "You showed up so you may as well put in the time and effort." What he meant by this is to not just go through the motions. Think of the steps I went through to get there. I set the alarm for 4am, got dressed, had a quick meal, drove 20 minutes to the Gym, worked out and then I drove twenty minutes home, showered, ate again — all before most people's days start. The point is, since you've gone through all this effort to be where you are, you may as well have specific effort while training (in practice or in chiropractic college). Don't just go through the motions.

Over the years, I've heard many of our professions leaders speak about intention during the adjustment; seeing the bone move in the specific direction you are delivering the force while at that same time seeing the patient's body healing and being whole. This can also be called present time consciousness.

From the first moment I heard this, I have practiced it with every adjustment I've delivered since. I do believe this is why we get people cleared and healed from chronic issues. Our intention is that healing is happening. By applying this to your practice and life you'll be amazed at the outcomes.

Donny Epstein, D.C.

It is vital to consider the difference between your objectives in care and your strategies. To achieve the extraordinary, your strategies must serve the higher order objectives of why you are in practice, why you care for someone, and the impact you must make for this person. Will this visit be consistent with what is possible for this individual as part of a higher calling of humanity?

The 8 Laws of Chiropractic Success

The adjustment of a subluxation, the technique used, and your assessment tools are all strategies to achieve or measure your outcome. What is your highest intention beyond all jargon, beyond your profession or beliefs or desires? How does your every interaction, application, and outcome line up with your professional intention for this person to achieve and assess for success?

Is your Intention from your very first to last contacts with your practice member about the benefit to yourself or your practice? If so there will not be enough energy to sustainably impact the practice member. Is it about the correction of subluxation, a thermal scan, the leg check, spinal curve, or other clinical findings? If so, this also limits the results in practice and the engagement of the individual. Please realize that your objective is different than your strategy. A higher objective adds more energy to you and through your entrained field to those you are serving.

What is the consequence of your care for the individual, his life, those he relates to, etc.?

Is your mindset about making people more comfortable first, adjusting vertebra, and improving health? Is your focus on helping them to make healthier choices and advancing in their lives? Are you adjusting lives, futures, and destinies? What about the notion of liberation? Liberation 'from' (a symptom or condition) requires and gives less energy than liberation towards (a vibrant and energized existence).

Each objective lives at a different level of energy and impacts in greater ways to organize intelligence into greater impact for the individual and the world. When you link the larger outcome with your chiropractic strategies you can deliver adjustments with that something extra!

Please consider your personal energy and efficiency when you consider your intention for that individual and the range of outcomes that you will consider to assess the effectiveness of your care. The coherence of your information and energy systems will create a quantum entanglement with the field of your practice member and increase your effectiveness. Focus your intent on a combination of your higher rational mind's clinical outcomes and the innate calling for that client and step up in service to this higher calling.

Reggie Gold, D.C.

If your intention is to put the bone where you think it "belongs," you're doomed to failure. You can't have a right action in response to a wrong intention. No, I shouldn't say that because you can, but it would be purely by accident. A person could trip over the curb and correct his own subluxation, but that's much less likely than the reverse, which is tripping over the curb and getting a subluxation.

There's no doubt that if your intention is the correction of vertebral subluxation, you will concentrate more on what you're doing. If you lack the intention and you get sloppy, then you're going to be effective less often than otherwise. Intention is important in that it makes you more careful with examining the spine and in putting in the right force in the right direction.

Tim Young, D.C.

I have spent countless hours reading, attending lectures, and engaging in very in-depth conversations with some of the professions greatest minds on understanding intention. I have even been told by college professors that intention has nothing to do with healing or success in chiropractic.

My conclusion after all these years, as I sit here today, is that your intention is the artist of your heart that created everything you receive. Intention is the connection between your heart and your mind and without it I feel you become a dog chasing your tail.

I once walked into my office and the song, "All You Need Is Love" by the Beatles popped Into my head. I really don't listen to the Beatles and I cannot remember the last time I heard that song. The chorus kept replaying in my mind, "All you need is

The 8 Laws of Chiropractic Success

love." I had sixty-two walk-ins that afternoon and ended up adjusting 142 patients in three hours. One of my busiest afternoons still to this day.

Whenever I feel like I'm off, or the office is off slightly, I replay that song. The artist takes over and it's a magical thing that happens between me and my patients. Intention is the artist of the art in chiropractic.

Armand Rossi, D.C.

Intention is the energy that goes along with your goals. Intention is that energy that follows through where you may not. For example, how many times have you told patients to lay on their right side when you actually meant left — and they laid on their left side anyway? Your intention got through even though your words did not.

If your intention is focused on your goal, you may make a negative statement like, "I'm tired today," but your intention will push you forward anyway. The intention is the important part in that it can overcome mental or verbal resistance.

Jessica Harden, D.C.

Intention is defined as what a person has in mind to create for a specific future outcome. Just by definition alone, intention by itself cannot create anything. It always requires action.

Ask yourself, "What is my intention in what I say or do?" Are you going through the motions or do you have a destination for what you put out? Words and actions will go to waste if intention is absent.

I have often heard it said that if you don't pick your direction or vision it will be chosen for you. Thus, if you lack intention with your actions or words, the person receiving them may be the person choosing where that conversation or interaction goes. You should always be leading your patients and never reacting.

The 8 Laws of Chiropractic Success

Think about when you are educating a patient on chiropractic and ask yourself, "Am I going through the motions?" Are you truly trying to connect and guide this person? That small step can drastically change the outcome of your results.

Look at an archer's training. How much skill goes into aiming and prepping the arrow versus the physical action of letting go? The aim and preparation are the most important aspects when hitting the target. If you release your actions and words without a specific direction, how can you be upset if you miss the intended target? Take ownership of intentionally preparing and mastering your actions so you can consistently hit your target.

Jason Deitch, D.C.

A person's intention is a person's aim or plan. Understanding and being conscious of your aim or plan drives your daily attitude and actions. If your intention is to "serve" as many people in your community as you can, then you will behave differently than if your intention is to "get" as many new patients as you can.

People most often think about one's intentions when it comes to a relationship. You ask yourself, "What is this person's intentions with this relationship?" Well, that's exactly what people are asking themselves about their relationship with you and your practice. What is this chiropractor's intentions? When you make care plan recommendations for people, they wonder, "Is this doctor recommending this care because it's what's best for my health or because it's what's best for their income?"

Being clear on your intentions drives your energy, your communication style, and your office policies.

Being clear on your intentions drives your energy, your communication style, and your office policies. It's an invisible force that people will be listening for, whether you're aware of it or not.

The 8 Laws of Chiropractic Success

The most successful people in the world have clear intentions within themselves, which manifest in their daily lives. It impacts how they prioritize themselves, their family, staff, patients, clients and community. It's essential to be self-aware enough to be conscious of your intentions. Then make sure you're communicating your intentions clearly with all of the people in your life.

Claudia Anrig, D.C.

Vision is seeing where you want to go; intentions are how you're going to get there. Perhaps for you it's a game plan and the premeditated steps you'll take to fulfill your vision.

The intention part is the realization that you're now going to take the necessary actions to fulfill your dreams and outline the steps needed to get there.

Neil Cohen, D.C.

We often hear the words, "What you think about you bring about." Depending on its application, intention is either a powerful tool or it is not. When you say, "I can't" you'll be correct 100% of the time. Dr. Sid Williams mentored many who declared, "I CAN, I WILL, and I MUST!" The combination of this affirmation along with a determined mindset and strategic action steps yields successful intention.

Oftentimes our intent is to say and do things yet they just never quite happen. What I want you to understand is what often takes place is exactly what your intentions are. I know for some of you that statement can sting - only if you have excuses.

When the chiropractor declares, "My intention was to get at least ten new patients at the screening but I only got three," or "My intention was for each new patient to bring their spouse to the x-ray and financial report but no one complied," it was not their intention to get ten new patients or to have spouses attend the meeting. Their attention was not on their intention. If it was, they would have achieved what they were determined to achieve 100% of the time.

You always get your desired intention when it is backed by determination. When that is missing then it is nothing more than wishful thinking to achieve your coveted goal.

When you're missing your "intended" mark, do a real gut check, take self-inventory, and don't kid yourself. Ask the questions, "Am I determined enough, am I committed enough, where is my attention, and what is my true intention?"

Gerard Clum, D.C.

Intention is the variable that makes things work. You either have a default intention or you have an active, deliberate intention. Either way, it's going to play a role in everything you do. Whether it's saying good morning to your spouse, dealing with a patient, or passing a homeless guy on the street, the intention you bring to each exchange (and to your life) is paramount.

If you intend to live a life of service or to live your life from a position of abundance, then opportunities for the demonstration of that intention begin to present themselves. If you don't have a conscious intention in life, you're just moving along with the flow of the stream. You'll get battered against the bottom once in a while and you'll get battered against the sides now and then. You'll also pop up to the top and get a sight of the surface before the next ebb and flow cycle takes you right back down with the current.

Vision is what gives you a rudder to control your progress

> **You either have a default intention or you have an active, deliberate intention. Either way, it's going to play a role in everything you do.**

in the flow and helps draw people to you who can be served by your vision. Your intention makes it all work.

Liam Schubel, D.C.

Intention is probably one of the most misunderstood words in the chiropractic profession. In the technique world you can clearly see chiropractic students and chiropractors that feel intention is hugely important to the successful chiropractic adjustment. I disagree. Consequence is much more important than intention as it relates to the adjustment.

As an example, take someone who has a vertebral subluxation at C1. I can intend all I want to correct that C1 vertebral subluxation and unless I have the technical skills and clear objective measures to know the consequence of my actions, then I will not achieve the results no matter how well intentioned I have been.

Where intention does play a key role in your clinical outcomes is in how that intention is expressed in your non-verbal communication. Aside from your adjusting skills, the practice member's faith in the doctor has been shown to play a key role in the practice member's clinical outcome. When you set your intention to loving the practice member and achieving the objective of chiropractic, (Location, Analysis and Correction of Vertebral Subluxation) that intention is non-verbally communicated to the practice member.

Just before I enter any interaction with a practice member I focus on my intention. "I love you and I can help you." It is that message that is being transmitted to the practice member that creates a greater clinical outcome. It is an intention that elicits certainty and trust in the eyes and hearts of the practice member. All successful chiropractic practices have doctors whose intentions elicit trust and certainty from their practice members.

The 8 Laws of Chiropractic Success

Daniel & Richelle Knowles, D.C.'s

Where intention meets mindset; vision, action, skill, love, service, and magic happen. The more you refine your intention with that extra something, the more magic will be delivered and experienced within your results. Take a car for instance. It can be used for multiple things. It can be used for travel, it can be used for entertainment, and oddly enough, a vehicle can even be used as a murder weapon. All of these are the potential outcomes of the act of driving. The difference is in the intention of the driver.

For you to have the best journey as a chiropractor you must make sure to hone your intentions with the greatest clarity. The greater the clarity, the more enjoyable and fruitful the journey will become for you and most importantly your passengers; those "souls on board" that you're graciously caring for.

In fact, a more honed intention will make up for less than ideal action, less than ideal mindset, less than ideal systems, less than ideal vision, and less than ideal service. However, the best results will always come from the optimization of all of these.

Is it possible for you to have a less clear intention and enjoy the ride as much as your passengers? Absolutely! However, to experience the greatest journey, to have the most outcomes in the shortest amount of time, and to impact the most lives, your intention must line up perfectly with all of your other assets — thus creating miracles.

Lou Corleto, D.C.

Intention is paramount. One error that many health care practitioners make (and I want to stress that I don't believe we should have ever been included in the health care model because we're a life model) is in defining their intentions. For instance, a practitioner's intention for a cancer patient might be to have that person get well and stay on the planet with his or her loved ones. But what if that isn't the intention of the individual on a higher level? What if his or her time is up and it's time to go home?

The 8 Laws of Chiropractic Success

It really is important for practitioners to get clear on what their intentions are. We can have compassion but we have to realize that compassion can get in the way. What is our intention when we're communicating the chiropractic message? Is it to empower? Is it to control? What is our intention when making that adjustive thrust? Is it to set a person free? Is it to treat a person so his or her back pain and migraine goes away? What's your intention?

CJ Mertz, D.C.

John C. Maxwell gave the world the phrase, "Fail forward fast." I think intention is really about not *trying* to do something. Absolute failure is to have the mindset of just *trying* to do something. In the movie "Star Wars," Yoda says, "Don't try, do!" I think that's the essence of intention.

The intent is not "trying" to do something. It's as if you notice a child chasing a ball who's about to run in front of a car coming down the street. You don't *try* to run out there and save that child. You do whatever it takes and don't even think about it.

Intent is doing whatever it takes to reach your goal. Since you're not simply trying, you have the right to fail and make mistakes. A huge part of success is skinning your knees and getting back up.

Intent gives us the freedom to make mistakes, and to learn and grow from them. If we really understand that we can "fail forward fast," we'll have the freedom to take more actions, risks, and stretch ourselves. Intent is the will to do rather than the will to try.

Thom Gelardi, D.C.

Intention has to be translated into action. An intelligent intention that benefits you, your practice members, and community is a good starting place. Intentions need to be backed up with competence, desire, and the proper use of your resources. Intention as a mystical, magical wand has never appealed to me.

The 8 Laws of Chiropractic Success

Patrick Gentempo, D.C.

Intention is the motion that follows vision. I have a vision of something that I want to accomplish and now I have an intention to make it happen. If you're unclear about your intentions or if your actions contradict them, you fail.

Christopher Kent, D.C.

Intention plays a tremendous role. There is a growing body of research to show that intent is a very important part of the healing process and that what the patient expects and what the doctor feels can be delivered are very, very important.

It is absolutely essential to have the right positive intent. What should that intent be? That intent should be seeing the perfection of that individuals manifestation. If you have that vision, all of the bad stuff goes away. When you see people as perfectly manifesting their humanity and you're thinking about and focused on that, you don't get into other problems.

What are you thinking about when they're on the table? Are you thinking, "What a cutie?" Are you thinking, "Let's talk about sports or the weather?" When you have all of that other junk floating around, you can't clear your mind, you can't have that pure and honorable intent, which the patient will absolutely feel. Once you get in that state, everyone loves it.

Larry Markson, D.C.

Intention plays a major role in *everything*. In fact, "The Power of Intention," one of the great works by Wayne Dyer, talks about this at great length. What is your intention? My intention is simply to help as many people as I can. The power of intention gives you the power of focus and concentration; it's a mind-target which zeroes you in.

You must have an intention more than mere survival. Many

chiropractors just show up in survival mode. My intention is to change the neighborhood and community, ultimately changing the way they think. My intention is to help change the way that people think so they can express boundless success and happiness.

Jeanne Ohm, D.C.

Your intention determines what you will manifest. That's why you have to expand your intention and continuously re-evaluate it. Ask yourself if what you're doing is true to who you really are — or is it simply about making bucks? Sure, you have to make a living but is that your primary intention, or are you truly doing what you do to be part of a shift in consciousness? Let's align our intentions with consciously being part of that shift.

Tedd Koren, D.C.

Intention plays a part clinically as well as in life. It's always been known that your intention can change the world. However, it's absurd to think that if you have a good intent you can "fix" your patients no matter what technique you use. All doctors want their patients to get better but some doctors do a better job at it than others. It's not necessarily intent; it's that they work their asses off to develop good procedures, know what they are doing, and study real hard.

Just having a fluffy feeling that you want people to get better isn't enough.

Just having a fluffy feeling that you want people to get better isn't enough. You have to actualize it and make it real. Believing, hoping, and wishing isn't enough in order to repair the world, which is our job. We have to always remember to do good deeds, be charitable, teach, and educate ourselves and others. Our role is as teacher and educator and that's where our intention needs to be.

The 8 Laws of Chiropractic Success

Terry A. Rondberg, D.C.

I think intention is critical to success in chiropractic and all aspects of business and life. It's one thing to know where you want to go, and another to know how you're going to get there. Intention is like having a map or GPS. B.J. Palmer, D.C. once said something to the effect that you don't take the train to one city when you want to get to someplace else. You have to look at the schedule, make choices, and form the true intention to proceed to your goal.

It's just as important to have clear intention as it is to have a vision.

It's just as important to have clear intention as it is to have a vision. The vision is the mental picture of your destination; intention is the strong inner knowledge that you will get there as well as your precise plan as to how you'll make the journey. The two go hand in hand.

Joe Strauss, D.C.

Intention has to do with continually focusing on your vision and the different ways you can fulfill that vision. Personally, I always accepted the idea that the body runs and heals itself, and that our job as chiropractors is to allow that expression to take place by correcting subluxations.

Once I set my intention to communicating that concept to every person I came in contact with, my practice truly became successful. My intention was to get the message out, not hold it in.

I know chiropractors who can talk about philosophy very clearly, but they don't communicate it to other people. I could sit and talk about Innate Intelligence with these doctors but, unfortunately, they never shared any of these ideas with their patients or others and never brought them down to the level that the public could understand. The intention of helping everyone understand about the true purpose of chiropractic is a key to success in your practice and all your endeavors.

The 8 Laws of Chiropractic Success

Arno Burnier, D.C.

Intention is vital in the adjustment but it's also vital in all areas of interaction with people in our offices. Regarding the adjustment, however, your entire office will reflect your intention — whether it's aggressive, loving, caring, supportive, or whatever. That intention comes through in all areas of who you are and what your office environment is like.

John Demartini, D.C.

Whatever is highest in your hierarchy of values is where your maximum attention, maximum retention of information, and maximum intention are. Any time you place a high value on something, your intention is going to be very intense and powerful there. That's why you want to make sure that your real highest value is on building a practice. If you do, you will have your intention there and you will manifest there.

Your intention dictates your actions, what you see in the world, and the opportunities you take advantage of. Without question, the power of intention and creation are keys.

D.D. Humber, D.C.

Regarding intention, Webster says, *"to aim, plan, firmly fixed or directed upon an object; earnest, seditious."* Every self-help book I have ever read has always stressed the importance of planning. If you are serious about reaching your goals in life, laying out a specific and detailed plan on how to reach that goal is essential.

To the Chiropractic student and to the Chiropractor, planning and goal setting is a must. To the student, it begins with planning and preparing to pass exams, always having the goal of graduating with a D.C. degree and ultimately beginning a lifetime of service as a Chiropractor.

Having been personally involved for over half a century in Dr. Sid Williams' Dynamic Essentials Seminars, as well as spending almost twenty-five years in Chiropractic education, I can say without any reservation, that all success I have witnessed came from individuals who planned extensively. Just as baking a cake begins with a recipe, so becoming successful in school and in practice first begins with a plan.

Chuck Ribley, D.C.

The power of intention is the way in which I move forward into dream. Power of intention is based on two factors; focus and believability. First, FOCUS means I could not move forward unless I am living in the NOW. PRESENT TIME CONSCIOUNESS is the key to focus.

Second is BELIEVABILITY. One has to be able to believe in the effectiveness of chiropractic health and also in the ability to have a sustainable practice. The friends I associated with and the books I read are some of the things that permitted the believability in chiropractic and also to build the successful practice I had.

∞

Ross McDonald and Rebecca Vickery, D.C.'s

Intention is a key component to success. Richard Branson frequently states, "Success comes from living with an intent and a purpose." Intention is the link between writing goals and achieving them through action. It is the part of the interaction with another person where you take responsibility for the actions you are taking and the outcome of that action.

Intention is an energy, a field of endless possibilities which can be influenced by focus, presence, and gratitude. If your intention is to be successful and help many on their path to health, you will achieve that. Being clear on your intention is crucial to success. If you are unsure of what you are doing and why you are doing it, your patient interaction will be unsuccessful on a variety of levels.

The 8 Laws of Chiropractic Success

Sharon Gorman, D.C.

When I am delivering the sacred chiropractic adjustment I think of intention. When I adjust someone, my intention is to reconnect them with their source; removing interference to their fullest expression of life. At that moment in time, I don't think they understand that, but that is what is in my head and heart. They are thinking they want to get rid of something (pain) and I'm thinking I want them to give them something (life). I typically will not say that to them because they are not ready to hear it and it might turn them off. Still, that is my intention.

On their first visit, my intention is to do or say whatever I can so they understand chiropractic enough to want to be a patient under regular care, along with their families, for the rest of their lives. If I directly told them this when they first entered the practice, because they have an ache or pain, they would have run for the hills.

I slowly court them over time and build trust. I don't want them to think I want them to change everything they understand about life and health on their first visit. If I did, they would probably never come back. I wouldn't have had the chance to take them through the process of choosing to bring their family in and make an informed decision about their health.

Most people aren't used to making the choice that I'm intending for them to make so I walk beside them and make my case. The longer I've been in practice, the better I've become at converting people to a chiropractic lifestyle. I live by example, showing them how to think from the inside-out rather than from the outside-in. My intention is always there, I meet them where they are at, and I never make them wrong.

Sometimes your intentions do not need to be voiced. They can live in your heart and quietly guide your actions.

Brian Kelly, D.C.

Two chiropractors delivering what appears to be the exact same spinal adjustment, at the same spinal level, will have completely different results on their patients. For some D.C.'s, as they are adjusting patients, it appears as though time stops; where they become a vessel for energy to flow from the Universe through them. Others discuss the stock market activity, weather, and sports as they are adjusting their patients, not connected to the universal energies whatsoever.

As you raise your energy and vibration, you will increase the vibration and energy in your patients. For other D.C.'s, their intention may be limited to only increasing range of motion and decreasing pain. Neither is good or bad or right or wrong. The question remains, what is your intention?

Perhaps Albert Einstein said it most eloquently, "Everything is energy and that's all there is to it. Match the frequency of the reality you want and you cannot help but get that reality. It can be no other way. This is not philosophy, this is physics."

Kevin Jackson and Selina Sigafoose-Jackson, D.C.'s

When a new patient enters our office our intention has never been, and will never be to "close them," "sign them up," or anything from a self-serving standpoint. Our pure intention is to do a detailed chiropractic assessment, a detailed doctor's report (explanation of chiropractic), and a detailed specific chiropractic adjustment.

Our intention is to try and allow a patient to get a glimpse of what the chiropractic philosophy is all about, allow them to experience a chiropractic adjustment, and then allow them to make their own decision about chiropractic at our office.

When an established patient comes in for an office visit our intention is to connect the neurological loop between the brainstem and the cells of their organs and muscles. The intention is never to "get" anything from the patient — it's only to "give."

∞

The 8 Laws of Chiropractic Success

Jim Dubel, D.C.

On a daily basis I try to reach as many people as possible through Chiropractic. Every conversation begins with me introducing myself as a Doctor of Chiropractic. In some way, shape, or form I explain what Chiropractic is and how it would improve the health of the person I am speaking to.

Just think, if every person I introduce chiropractic to "gets the idea" and starts care with myself or another Chiropractor, I have changed their life forever.

Amanda and Jeremy Hess, D.C.'s

Intention is a "super power" for those who know how to use it in a positive and life-giving way. There are so many examples of things we all do in our lives that when the "act" vs. the "intention" is varied, the outcome is vastly different or affected.

Let's look at the example of two people having a glass or two of wine. One is enjoying the taste, texture, or the vintage, while the other is just trying to forget about a bad day at work. The act of drinking the wine is the same but the intention is totally different and therefore so is the outcome.

Regarding intention and chiropractic practice, the action or force given with an adjustment might be the same with two chiropractors, yet ones intention is to free the spine of vertebral subluxation and restore life, while the other is intending to simply decrease inflammation and pain. The intention going into the adjustment (or anything else in life) greatly determines the outcome of the action itself.

The growth or stagnation of a chiropractic office is very dependent on the intention of the chiropractor and the team members level of functioning in that office. During the evaluation and initial education process, is the intention to get the potential new practice member out of pain as soon as possible, focus all education towards pain relief, and recommend pain reduction techniques OR are we moving the practice member's mindset towards an understanding of the cause of the problem being vertebral subluxation and educate them towards a longer-term approach of health revitalization through ongoing corrective and maintenance chiropractic care?

Intention is a choice we must make or our selfish human nature will likely lead towards negative outcomes and disappointing let downs. Check yourself and check your intentions on what you routinely do. Observe how you interact with people and what your intentions are when caring for them in your practice. When you focus your intentions in a positive and willful manner, you'll be surprised at how your entire life dramatically changes.

Chapter 4

"The best way to find yourself is to lose yourself in the service of others." — Mahatma Gandhi

Law Four – Service

David K. Scheiner, D.C.

When was the last time you took a long walk alone? Was it in the city? Was it in nature on a hike in the woods or on the beach? Did you get completely absorbed in the walk and lose track of time? Did you take a moment to observe everything your sight could take in; a visual impression of the terrain? There's something magical occurring when you take walks alone and lose yourself in the moment; becoming completely absorbed in the surroundings.

Being of service is the same thing. When you love what you do and do what you love, you are delivering and serving up Universal gifts to others. You are merely an empty vessel being used by God to deliver magic to his children. There's no ego involved and you have to quite literally move yourself aside in order for this wonderful exchange of energies to occur.

If you find yourself uptight and tense in your place of service you may want to re-evaluate what you are serving, who you are being of service to, and how you are getting in the way. To truly be of service you must be your authentic and genuine selves. Take an inventory of all the ways of behaving and acting in your life that are inauthentic to yourself and others. What's it costing you? You have to get really present to it or it will repeat over and over in your life, preventing you from being able to serve others at the highest levels possible. There's something to discover for yourself here, that if you're willing to look, can have you grow yourself and your business infinitely.

There is a magic in service that allows you and the receiver to be completely present. It directly relates to the intention of what you are giving your service for, coupled with how you are going about the delivery. Both the giving and the receiving of the service need to be gentle and passive in order for the loving service to have its positive healing effects. It also takes a certain amount of passion and a completely split open heart in order that each encounter you make has its wondrous intended outcome. With service, there's transformation that must show up as illogical in order for the magic healing effects to occur.

Cathy Wendland-Colby, D.C.

Muhammad Ali said, "Service to others is the rent you pay for your room here on earth."

Every one of you have amazing life changing stories to share, and you should share them. Do you know what you should realize in those precious stories? It ain't about you. It's about them and their connection with Innate. Sure, you facilitated the transformation by adjusting them and removing the interference, but when you detach from the outcome, you recognize it's never been about you. You provided a service, and while I truly believe it's the most important service available, their body accepted the adjustment and responded accordingly.

It's not about you or me. We are simply servants of the principle and merely a vessel. As Dr. Sid said, "A hollow weenie." Universal Intelligence flows from above, down, inside, and out through our hands to the people we are responsible for. Whether they're young or old, fit or fat, healthy or sick, rich or poor. Whether they "believe" in Chiropractic or you are their last ditch

The 8 Laws of Chiropractic Success

effort and whether they paid in full or are on a financial hardship — it's always about serving the principle, by serving the people.

There is no higher purpose in life than service. The way you serve more people is by getting out of your own way, opening your mouth, and educating people. Detach yourself from the outcome and remember; What we do for ourselves dies with us. What we do for others is eternal.

Clear your headspace before you walk into your office. It's go-time and your patients are trusting you to serve their families.

Jim Dubel, D.C.

Believe me, there are mornings I would like to lay in bed and get an extra hour of sleep but as a Chiropractor there is much work to be done, we still only see a very small percentage of the population. The oath that we take to serve humanity is one that requires vigilance.

There is no time off when you are a Chiropractor. You literally must be "on" 24/7. You never know when something you think, say, or do will affect the life of another individual.

∞

Neil Cohen, D.C.

Service is a heart centered attribute. Self-service is ego centric. Motives are only known by the Maker of men and the man himself. The greatest among men and women, whether chiropractor or student, are the ones who serve sacrificially. For the practitioner, this does not mean you don't get paid. Quite the contrary, it demonstrates that you've developed the habit of being empathetic, responsible, warm, caring, friendly, and purpose-filled.

Servants are not slaves; they have developed into great masters of listening, being hospitable, and are always on the lookout to lend a hand. They go the extra mile whenever they are afforded the opportunity.

Service is a skillset that you ought to compel yourselves to learn as quickly as possible. Money brings happiness and the serv-

The 8 Laws of Chiropractic Success

ice brings joy. Lacking the service-oriented heart will leave you in a quid pro quo or "this for that" mentality throughout your life.

"What's in it for me?" is not a heart centered question. The greatest question an authentic servant can ask is, "What's in it for them?" Do not turn Chiropractic into merely your career. Rather, like a seedling, water it, feed it, and nurture it into your beautiful calling as you go forth and serve humankind!

Tim Young, D.C.

Service in chiropractic is the WHY in chiropractic. When I am coaching a young chiropractor, the first question I ask them is, why are you adjusting this patient in the first place. I typically get any number of answers. When I keep digging I can usually lead them to the reasons that they were not even aware of; one being Service.

This is why the universe chose each particular individual and led them to this amazing profession. Service to every human that is alive is your chosen occupation. I believe very strongly that it was chosen for you. It is now up to you to deny or deliver on that choice.

Chuck Ribley, D.C.

Kahlil Gibran, in his book **The Prophet** said, "Work is love made visible and if you cannot work with love but only with distaste, it is better that you should leave your work and sit at the gate of the temple and take alms of those who work with joy." This explains the importance for me as a chiropractor; I love what I do.

In my 60 years in the chiropractic profession I always awaken in the morning with a desire to make the world a better place through chiropractic. Whether that's in the office or outside the office.

Jessica Harden, D.C.

It is not as much about providing a service with perfection as much as it is about the ongoing push to consistently deliver a service with a spirit of excellence. Joshua Medcalf, well known speaker and advisor, often writes about falling in love with the process. He explains that if you consume yourself in the training of an action, the delivery will be automatic and the result will take care of itself.

Often times, when your service is not producing the results you desire, you assume you need to change that service. In reality, you should be looking at how to get better at that service. The service is not only the adjustment; it is also the analysis, the customer service, and the connections made to encourage your patients on their healing journey. When you continually work to improve each aspect of your service they will each work for the other much like a finely tuned engine.

You should continually examine the service you provide for your patients and do the same with the service you provide for your team. Your team is one of (if not) the biggest investments in your practice. The team should never be viewed as an expense. I have heard it said, "If you raise up your team correctly, they should make you money and not cost you money." Your team sees a patient twice as often as the doctor; on the way in and on the way out. Think of how many heart connections could be made or how many TIC talks could be shared. Your team should be leading your patients on their health journey; building strong rapport and relationships with the patient.

Make sure to serve your team members well if you want them with you for the long journey. Learn how they like to be appreciated, continually remind them of your support, and create a culture where they can openly be creative. If you can create an experience in your office that embodies service with excellence, it will bring forth trust and commitment from your patients and team.

∞

Billy DeMoss, D.C.

Service is the action of aiding others. It's all about doing unto others as you would have them do unto you. I also believe that in practice, you have to raise the bar exponentially and deliver the highest level of service.

The 8 Laws of Chiropractic Success

At my practice we strive to give each patient the Ritz Carlton experience. Fortunately, we've been able to achieve it. From a warm greeting the moment they step into the office, to the decor and cleanliness; service is ever-present and all encompassing. That's probably one of the biggest attributes we have here at DeMoss Chiropractic — we deliver at a higher level than anywhere else.

We focus a lot on education and always provide more than what a patient expects within every aspect of service. Along their journey we're slowly educating them about chiropractic. Doctor means teacher and as a doctor of Chiropractic it's important that I deliver adjustments and educate the entire family on every component of total health.

∞

Jason Deitch, D.C.

A dedicated focus on "Service" is the backbone of success. Throughout history, mentors, teachers, preachers, authors, experts and success guru's all point to a deep passion for being of service to others as the key to unlocking a successful and fulfilling life.

Being of service to others is the one common denominator towards success taught across all cultures...

If you want to attract more new patients, then have a commitment to being of service to others. If you want to earn more money, then have a commitment to being of service to others. If you want more significance in life, then have a commitment to being of service to others. Being of service to others is the one common denominator towards success taught across all cultures and generations.

It's easy to feel entitled. It's common to feel like you deserve more. It's frustrating to not experience the level of success you see for yourself. Yet, when you take a step back and analyze what needs to happen to improve your life, business, or income, it's safe to say that reinvigorating your passion to be of service to others is the one simple solution that works time and time again.

The 8 Laws of Chiropractic Success

Guy Riekeman, D.C.

I have to distinguish between service and martyrdom. I'm not a big altruist, based on my (Ayn) Randian background. An altruist looks at the old communist manifesto model, "From each according to his ability, to each according to his need." This implies that if I have something, I have a responsibility to give it to somebody else. But I don't! If it's my idea, I have the right to keep my idea if I want to keep my idea, sell my idea, or whatever I do with my idea.

Service is about becoming the best I can become, because until I am the best I can become, I have nothing to offer humanity anyway. I serve humanity in a way that also serves me. You receive through the same hole you give through. The more you give, the more you're going to receive. I don't give in order to receive, but I know that I can't receive unless I give.

At Life University, there's a great quote over every door when you walk out of the Center for Chiropractic Education: "To Give, To Serve, To Love, and To Do out of a sense of abundance."

We are privileged human beings in this country and privileged human beings as chiropractors. Out of that sense of abundance you have to Give, Serve, Love, and Do. I actually teach a four-hour class to first-year students on the seven principles of giving and that's the first one: you give through the same hole that you receive through.

Frederick A. Schofield, D.C.

Viktor Frankl said, *"Find meaning in life by doing the work you want to do, and do it to distraction."* Starting your own practice is not something you rush into or take lightly as it has to be done more than just vaguely. So you should analyze the first part of your practice, and when you doubt, rely on your 7 great friends:

Who, What, Where, Why, When, Which, and How.
Patient Service has to do with patients trusting your Clinic. Love builds a clinic. Service feeds a clinic.

The 8 Laws of Chiropractic Success

3 Keys to Patient Service:

1) Welcome patients to your clinic:

   "Welcome Ms. Jones. It is our pleasure to have you as a patient." The welcome must be genuine and said with integrity. B.J. Palmer, D.C. said, "How do you measure success? RESULTS."

2) Compliance — is the patient congruent with the Dr.? Are we on the same page?

3) Gratitude:

   "Thank you for choosing our office. Spread the Word. Keep the Faith. Check you Monday"

Simple — Concise — Serve

Be Still and Sow and SO IT IS!!!

Teri and Stu Warner, D.C.'s

It has been said that the best way to find yourself is to lose yourself in the service of others. Everyone has a purpose in life and a talent to share. As chiropractors, our calling is unique and noble. We have the amazing opportunity to share our gift with the world. When we serve right, something special happens. On your busiest days serving the most people, you somehow find yourself filled with boundless energy. By anyone else's standards you should be exhausted. There is a fantastic energetic exchange between you and your patients that creates an increase!

Service is at the root of all we do. Walt Disney said it best, "Do what you do so well that they will want to see it again and bring their friends." This is a great principle for us all to strive for. Create an office environment where your patients enjoy their experience so much that they return time and time again, refer in their friends and family, and gladly pay for the experience. This level of service should inspire you and be your goal.

As graduates of Life Chiropractic College (now Life University), the fundamental guiding principle of the Lasting Purpose:

To Give, To Do, To Love, To Serve – out of our own abundance was instilled in us by Dr. Sid E. Williams. He taught us to have a willingness and desire to serve our community and our fellow man. We were also taught to have our sole focus be on a separate 'Service Hand' and 'Business Hand' when we are taking care of our patients. Although you need to do both, the two 'Hands' must remain separate and distinct.

Creating a patient-focused service culture with lots of "little extras" to set your office apart from others, is an opportunity that should not be missed. Since our office is maternity and pediatric focused, we've included special features to make our new mama's, baby's, and kids feel very special. We have a nursing chair, changing station with extra diapers and wipes, organic snacks, spring water, organic teas, and several toddler and kids play areas.

To give real service you must add something which cannot be bought or measured with money, and that is sincerity, integrity, and love. Make your office extra special by raising your level of service, and success is sure to follow!

∞

Donny Epstein, D.C.

I believe true service is about providing care for the sake of the person more than for your own benefit. It is care that goes beyond a practice member's symptoms or difficult circumstances and towards serving a person's highest calling. It is the spiritual intelligence which connects you and your client to what is really true, beyond conditioning of culture or mind.

It is in the wake of true service, service that often brings massive instability to one's conditioned and educated life, that your practice member hears Innates calling. Be it a whisper or a shout, below the conscious mind, to the conscious mind, or to the beyond rational mind — the calling is recognized. When service for the sake of service is rendered, there is an innate refinement in the care you provide, the words you speak and don't speak, and a resulting deepened sense of intimacy experienced by all involved in the healing experience.

The 8 Laws of Chiropractic Success

Daniel & Richelle Knowles, D.C.'s

Jim Parker, founder of Parker College of Chiropractic, coined the statement, "Loving service, my first technique." As a chiropractor, you are first and foremost operating in a service-based industry compared to retail or selling a product. You're there to serve people at a high level.

The definition of service is: The action of helping or doing work for someone. By focusing on another's needs first, you will always have more than enough. I remember a particular time when my family and I were going away for vacation on an exciting trip to Mexico. It was very early in the morning as we headed for the airport. Leaving at 4:00 AM for the flight was brutal on everyone and I was especially cranky.

When we got to the airport, the sky cap who helped us with our bags, was extremely smiley, chipper, and happy. This gentle and kind soul was going to be moving, shuffling, and loading luggage all day. In all of the service-related industries I've encountered, I have never met anybody more positive than he was. He was so genuinely happy to be of service to our family and from the looks of it, was far happier and more joyful than I was — and I was going to Mexico! I often think of this experience as I enter my office to make sure I load my heart up with the same service, vibration, and tone.

Service is not bound to any one industry, it's a state of being that is contagious and can shift the mood of the people you are working with. Be in a state of service first, and your work will be more appreciated.

Liam Schubel, D.C.

One of the meditations I have always done is a very easy yet powerful one. I spend ten minutes in meditation daily, thinking about this one question:

How can I serve more people?

Then I go on to mediate on this next question:

How can I serve the people that I am already serving...better?

The 8 Laws of Chiropractic Success

People who do business with me are always amazed that I have a tendency to get whatever I want in the business deals that I set up. The reason for this is that my mindset is constantly focused on how I can serve others. If I can just figure out how to serve other people in a high quality fashion and get them exactly what they want, then I will never have a problem getting what I want. The question becomes – what do YOU want?

A doctor of chiropractic is only as valuable as the quantity of service they provide as well as the quality of that service. A chiropractor cannot make an abundant life for themselves without serving others. The *only* way to make it to the top in the chiropractic profession is through serving others period. The key to fulfillment and joy as a chiropractor and student is to fall in love with the serving.

I once listened to an interview with a famous comedian. He was coming home to his apartment after being on the road for a while. As he was approaching the door to his apartment, his phone rang. He was informed that his wife had died in a tragic accident. At that very moment, two fans asked him to take "a selfie" with them. He made a decision to serve others instead of feeling sorry for himself. He stated that it was through service to others that he was able to heal himself. Whenever you want more in life look to serve more and do so at a higher level.

Kevin Jackson and Selina Sigafoose-Jackson, D.C.'s

Service is often such an overlooked idea in all forms of business. As chiropractors we feel incredibly passionate about customer service. All of our staff is standing all day long and ready to serve people. We train so that when any patient enters or leaves the building they are promptly greeted or said goodbye to.

Patients deserve the honor and dignity of being acknowledged of their importance. Everyone is special, especially the very unlikable and unlovable people. We are a service-driven industry with chiropractic being the vehicle. If there's one thing that stands out

The 8 Laws of Chiropractic Success

that we could teach a young practitioner, it's the art of service. Over delivering and over serving goes far beyond any conventional marketing program we've come across.

Sharon Gorman, D.C.

One of the core elements of being human is that we want to make a difference. When I am serving, I feel good about myself. When I share the chiropractic message with someone, I reflect on how it felt when someone first got that message through to me and I got the Big Idea. That is a very exciting moment and process to experience. As you know, the chiropractic philosophy isn't status quo (yet), so the more I talk to patients about it, the more real it becomes for me, and the tide slowly begins to turn as the patient understands this important message.

I love to get lost in service and some of my happiest moments are when I am practicing, not having time to think about my needs and wants. I am solely there to serve the patient. A patient doesn't care about our philosophy or office decor as much as whether we can help them. They want to know we care about them and when we are fully present with them, they know that they are the most important person in the world. Serve them well and make them feel truly special.

John Demartini, D.C.

If you're projecting what you think is important onto patients without caring enough to find out what their needs are and learn the art of communicating in the context of their values, there is no service.

Service is filling needs and respecting values of other people. Wise chiropractors encourage feedback to make sure they're communicating in accord with their patients' needs, values, and language. This allows them to provide greater service, which in turn creates greater practice growth, and wealth.

The 8 Laws of Chiropractic Success

Paul Reed, D.C.

Chiropractors are in the service business and naturally have giant giving hearts, wanting what's best for your patients. Having a giant service heart will build a giant practice, yet it is extremely important to remember to maintain balance between your service and business hands. I lost that balance about ten years into practice. I was so keenly focused on service and I found myself practically giving those services away. This continued for several months before I began feeling out of exchange and balance with our practice members.

I got caught in this trap and also believe other chiropractors can too. Having the natural desire to help coupled with the need to be liked, potentially exposes us to long-term failure. It is critical (I repeat), it is critical that you figure out your stop-loss and never operate below it. While a busy practice is fun and invigorating, the last thing you want to do is fill your practice up with practice members while not meeting your financial obligations.

Spend some thoughtful time evaluating and looking for your own unique sweet spot. What do I mean by this? Do the math and know exactly what your overhead is. Then calculate what your service fees must be in order for you to be profitable with the type of practice you desire. This is where practice becomes fulfilling and financially stable.

Lou Corleto, D.C.

Service is the root of intention. In that space of service, we are truly feeding others what they need in order to progress to their next level. Even though we think we know what that is, we don't.

When we're in a place of service, we're in humble gratitude to be there for individuals and to be the vehicle to assist them in receiving what they need in order to go to the next place in their process of life.

∞

The 8 Laws of Chiropractic Success

Reggie Gold, D.C.

Service plays a role in dedication. If I'm really concerned about correcting subluxation, I have at least pre-checked to see if a subluxation is there and I do what I think would possibly correct it and then — the most important thing of all — I post-check. Most chiropractors don't even bother to post-check, so how do they know if the subluxation has been corrected?

Chiropractors say to me, "How do you know if the subluxation is still there?" If you don't know that then how do you know it was there in the first place? The real art of chiropractic is to be able to identify the presence or absence of subluxation. Again, that's an art and not a science.

Brian Kelly, D.C.

From my own experience and observations of many, many chiropractors, the attitude of whether you are here to serve humanity or just see patients and make a living, will have a dramatic effect on two things. First, your reputation and second, the joy you find in your work.

The desire to serve fellow people is one of the highest callings you can have. Keeping this premise close to your heart and soul, you will always go the extra mile and love serving people.

When considering service within the context of a patients' experience in a chiropractic office, I am reminded of the words of the late poet Maya Angelou, "I've learned that people will forget what you said, people will forget what you did, but people will never forget how you made them feel."

Creating a healing environment and keeping your focus on a magical patient service experience will always attract people to your office, increase your patient retention, and have a dramatic impact on your clinical results.

∞

Thom Gelardi, D.C.

The chiropractor's work is all about service — to patients, the community, and the profession. Service begins with competence and competence incorporates great knowledge and skill. Almost anyone can be taught to move vertebrae. However, adjusting a vertebral subluxation is as different from merely moving a vertebra as pitching in the strike zone is from merely throwing a ball.

Service isn't measured in terms of time spent with a practice member or the amount of work done on the patient. Service lies in the careful analysis of the spine and the skillful adjustment of the offending vertebra.

Professionals, be they golfers, writers, or chiropractors, work with an economy of motion. A force needed to move the correct vertebra in the correct direction is far more of a service than the unneeded movement of eight vertebrae.

A valuable part of our service is teaching our practice members the principles of health. These principles have generally been called chiropractic philosophy, but they are universal principles that are important enough to be taught by most chiropractors.

Gerard Clum, D.C.

Service is central. There's always a service to be had. Whether it's to serve the best needs of chiropractors or the public, service will be had.

When you combine your vision with your intention and apply it in a spirit of service (or, as Sid [Williams] put it, "Loving for the sake of loving, giving for the sake of giving, and serving for the sake of serving") on some level it is an unencumbered reality.

We all know people who give to get and it works for a while. We also know individuals who give to live. Those who give to live have returns in ways that are hard to fathom and appreciate at times. It's the same with service. Asked to name a great person, some people might say Michael Jordan, others General Patton.

The 8 Laws of Chiropractic Success

More often than not, I think they're going to say Martin Luther King, Nelson Mandela, Mother Teresa, and others who've lived a life of service. We might erect a statue of a general but we quote, believe in, and reflect on the Mother Teresa's of the world.

Patrick Gentempo, D.C.

Chiropractic is a service business. Chiropractors need to keep in mind that they're dealing with consumers who have a limited amount of money but unlimited choices of what to spend it on.

> **You cannot be selfless and simultaneously derive the benefit of profits.**

They're not going to come to your office unless you have a very compelling reason for them to spend that money on you rather than something or someone else. You must provide an extraordinary service that individuals perceive is worth more than what they're spending.

A purely selfless act doesn't result in any benefits for you, including profits. You cannot be selfless and simultaneously derive the benefit of profits.

Unfortunately, many people get into the selfless server mindset — and they end up broke. The contradiction here is that they want to help more and more people but the fewer resources they have, the fewer people they *can* help.

What they need to achieve is a proper exchange of values by providing an extraordinary service for a very fair fee. When you put that model together you succeed.

Arno Burnier, D.C.

Service is a very crucial and essential ingredient. When you come from a place of service that's authentic and real, chiropractors experience joy, happiness, and fulfillment. These feelings spill over into every moment of your lives and practice, being felt and perceived — subliminally or consciously — by all the people you see or touch during the day.

The 8 Laws of Chiropractic Success

Claudia Anrig, D.C.

Service, whether it's giving a chiropractic adjustment or being kind to somebody on the street, is putting your vision and intention into action. Most people engaged in service aren't sitting up there on a pedestal expecting applause for what they do. They usually work quietly in the background but without them, you'd never have the great experience of having your meals served with a smile in the restaurant, or seeing a wonderful theatrical performance on stage. It's all thanks to those people behind the scenes.

Whenever I talk about service, my dad comes to mind. A quiet man — known to speak maybe three words in a week, yet a giant to everybody in his practice — his hands, intent, and focus spoke volumes. When I think about service, he certainly comes to mind.

∞

Joe Strauss, D.C.

The concept of service is directly related to knowing what we do, what we have, and recognizing the vital need for all humans to benefit from chiropractic.

Once you know what chiropractic is and how important it is for every man, woman, and child in the world, it just naturally follows that you want to make sure everyone — or at least as many people as you can possibly physically handle — receive chiropractic care. Why would you want to allow people in your community to walk around subluxated when you know how important it is to have those subluxations corrected?

Sometimes I tell my practice members, "I think chiropractic is so important to your life, health, and family that I would pay you to come in to my office."

Obviously, I can't do that so the next best thing is to give my services away. I really can't afford to do that either, so the third best thing would be to have a fee system that makes it available to every person. That's why I have a "box on the wall" practice. And since I know people's time is limited as well, my office is open 12 hours a day.

The 8 Laws of Chiropractic Success

We try to drop as many barriers as we can for people and they pick up on that. They think, "Wow, he must feel chiropractic is really important if he allows us to pay whatever is within our means and open such long office hours to make it convenient for us to come in."

I'm not saying everybody has to do this. It's just my way of demonstrating service to my community.

Tedd Koren, D.C.

Service directly ties into your vision and you live to serve and serve to live. You have a talent and a skill to go out there and teach and heal the world. It appears that when we just give with no hidden agenda, things seem to always come back to us. For some reason selfishness just doesn't work.

Terry A. Rondberg, D.C.

Service is one of the cornerstone principles of success. You need to be of service and to serve something greater than yourself. Sid Williams, D.C. used to say, "We are all just little weenies with a hole at each end searching for creature comforts."

Once you've satisfied your senses and acquired enough material stuff and aren't in desperate survival mode anymore, you begin to think about and want a higher purpose, something that involves service, and something greater than yourself.

Have a vision that's bigger than just you and satisfying your own needs. Have a vision of helping others. Have a vision of serving others and serving a greater power in your life.

I have a very clear vision that I'm not here simply for myself; I am here to serve. I serve a higher power than myself and do so by serving the people created by that greater power.

Whenever I bent over a patient to adjust an Atlas, I would always say a prayer to myself, "Lord, please help me and use me so that this person can become whole again spiritually and physically."

When I introduced a thrust using my educated mind as well as that little "extra special something" B.J. (Palmer) talked about, then I was out of the picture and just sat back and watched the results.

The universal power flowed through me and that person so that balance, harmony, and optimum health could be re-established. My intention was to always see that happen. Those moments with the application of the thrust are sacred moments, moments of grace, and moments of blessing because we are being used as a tool to make that happen. As soon as we get in the way everything gets screwed up.

∞

Armand Rossi, D.C.

Service takes you out of the ego and puts you in tune with the universe. Service and gratitude work hand in hand and gratitude even comes before service. The book, "The Science of Getting Rich," by Wallace Wattles talks about some of these principles. I suggest you read that book when you find the time.

∞

CJ Mertz, D.C.

I often tell clients, "Your procedures are your promotions and your promotions are your procedures." Restaurants, movie studios, and business marketing people know that word-of-mouth "advertising" can generate incredible street buzz. When people have a positive experience, they just have to tell others about it.

The same thing goes for chiropractors. The service you provide must be at a level where people simply *have* to tell other people about it.

That comes right back to the essence of the chiropractic purpose: to see that the message of chiropractic is spreading through the land. One of the greatest ways you can spread the message is to provide world-class service, the kind of service that makes people want to tell everyone else about their experience in your office and, of course, continue coming to you.

Because of the exceptional service you offer, not only do these people enjoy the lifetime benefits of chiropractic for themselves, but they help the chiropractic message spread like wildfire.

The 8 Laws of Chiropractic Success

Ross McDonald and Rebecca Vickery, D.C.'s

To truly be successful and live a legendary life, you must be in balance with all aspects of that life. One aspect of being in balance is being of service to others – it is as important to you as it is to the people you serve. When you constantly take from the world without giving back to it, it keeps you in a state of constant survival, a place of suspended animation where you are neither moving forward or backward.

Maslow's Hierarchy of needs helps us to understand the concept of service and success. To move from survival — through stability — to success and significance in our lives, it's mandatory that chiropractors focus on the needs of others; to focus on giving more to the people we serve. What service really comes down to is ethics, accountability, and responsibility to something bigger than we are. For you and I it's the people we serve in our practices.

∞

Janice Hughes, D.C.

Success is intimately tied in with service. To serve, to love, and to give. This is a standard that you will see throughout many world class and 5-star businesses. To serve the customer, to serve the client, and ultimately to serve your own business based on this incredible reputation within your community.

In Chiropractic, if you start with the focus on serving the person right in front of you, then all else follows. All too often you are focused on something that happened earlier in your day, or in the other extreme something that is going to happen in the future. Your fears, emotions, and worries get in the way of the person or situation that is right in front of you. Bluntly, this means there's a lack of true focus and attention on serving the person or situation that is right there.

Serve in the moment...and watch as the success pours in.

Starting from a premise to serve, truly opens the door to all the universal possibilities available to you. When you regularly come from this space, you tap into hidden resources you may not have even consciously known that you had.

The 8 Laws of Chiropractic Success

Larry Markson, D.C.

We get paid for the service we perform. Jim Parker, D.C., once said to me, "You have to have a compassion to serve much more than a compassion to survive." And right now, that is not happening in the chiropractic profession. I think we're servants. We're servants to the human body and we have to render loving kindness with great intent, which gives more to people than they pay in return.

It's my belief that if people pay you $50 for an adjustment, you must make certain that what you give them is worth more than that amount. That doesn't mean throwing in extras like therapies, a lollipop, or a cervical pillow to make up the difference! It means giving them more of you, more of your focus, more of your intention, and ultimately greater service.

D.D. Humber, D.C.

Receiving good service from others wherever you may be is always an uplifting and appreciated experience. A privately owned fast food restaurant that started out in my hometown of Atlanta, Georgia, "Chick-fil-a" trains all employees to respond to customers thusly: "My pleasure." This means, of course, that it was a pleasure to be of service to you. By the way, Chick-fil-a is now the third largest fast food restaurant in America. Good service is by no means found everywhere you go. In fact, we often find ourselves wondering where can we find good service!

Chiropractic students and Chiropractors alike should be well versed in the importance of courteous service. I have often heard the expression and believe it to be true, "The better the service, the better the success." It is my opinion that this certainly applies to Chiropractors. It is not uncharacteristic for young people to have the attitude "It is all about me." But as one matures it becomes evident that if we are to become successful, our thought pattern must be "It is all about others!" I believe from a spiritual perspective, setting our egos aside and committing ourselves to serving our fellow man is what our Creator intended for us to do.

Amanda and Jeremy Hess, D.C.'s

This law of service reminds us of a story which you may of heard before, yet it bears worth repeating...

There once was a very wise old king. He wanted to ensure his kingdom and way of life would continue after his time had expired. He called his most trusted and enlightened advisors to his chamber. He told them, "I want you to gather all the knowledge in the kingdom and bring it here to the castle where it can be found and enjoyed by every man, woman, and child from this time forward."

His best men were dispersed throughout the kingdom and were gone for many years. The day finally arrived when they began to show up at the gates. Wooden wagons were filled with books and papers stacked so high, the horses labored to move their weight. Wagon after wagon after wagon appeared.

When the King saw the accumulation filling the grand courtyard and spilling over into the streets and meadows beyond the castle wall, he again assembled his most trusted and enlightened advisors. This time he requested that they reduce the amount of material to only the essential. He ordered them to remove the duplicates, strike out inconsistency, and return with only what they knew to be true.

After several years, his advisors appeared with a collection of books nicely bound and numbered. Looking over the courtyard at this vast collection, the King grew saddened, for he knew this was still too much for one person to consume and understand. He pleaded once more that they refine the assortment of texts to the very essence of what they knew.

After a year of discarding, arranging, and organizing, his best scholars and scribes brought him one very large book. The relieved King thanked his men profusely but asked one last time that they condense this vast volume. He told them, "My wish is that any man, woman, or child of all persuasions and with all levels of education and understanding could open this book and receive the knowledge necessary to go through life.

And so it was, the King was presented with one book that

contained one page and on this one page read one word. And in this one word was the meaning of life.... SERVE. The King rejoiced.

Serving your Family, Practice members, and your Community through one simple yet sacrificial manner, Service...is the key to a successful practice and life. It seems so easy, yet it takes discipline and a continual renewing of the mind to serve the multitudes on a long-term basis.

Steve Judson, D.C.

Service for services sake delivered to others is the greatest gift we can give to mankind. No matter how much trial, tribulation, and heartache a day may bring, when you get lost in service your own spirit naturally heals, which aides in the healing of others and ultimately the planet.

When your so-called "needs" are removed from your consciousness, you won't desire for anything because you already have everything. Since you have everything, the focus must now shift from wanting to serving. Serve the masses and the universe will continuously serve you. Serve through chiropractic and watch the dreams of the world come true around you.

Brad Glowaki, D.C.

Everything from the words, the gestures, the office aromas, and the aesthetics, to your own physiology, play a part in the service you provide for your patients.

Said differently, the service you and your team provide creates the context for the adjustment. The context is more important than the content — it has the power to either add-to or take-away-from the healing process. For example, you cannot be in defense mode and be healing at the same time.

Be cognizant of and practice always with that in mind.

The 8 Laws of Chiropractic Success

Gilles LaMarche, D.C.

I had the privilege to meet Dr. James W. Parker while I was a 3rd year chiropractic college student in September 1977. From that day until his passing in 1997, I had the honor of receiving his mentorship. His major life mantra was "Loving Service — My First Technique." Dr. Parker exemplified that value and he had the amazing ability to transfer it to his mentees.

I took that mantra as my own and have since applied it to all aspects of my life; every relationship and every interaction. Later in life, I heard someone say, "Service is the price you pay for taking up space on this planet." In that moment, I understood the concept of fair exchange and crafted my personal purpose statement which I edited to become: *"I pledge my life to my greatest expression of love and service for the benefit of humanity."*

Yes, choosing to serve every day is fair exchange for the life we get to live. Two of my favorite service quotes are: "The best way to find yourself is to lose yourself in the service of others," and "To give real service you must add something which cannot be bought or measured with money, and that is sincerity and integrity." Always look for ways to serve others with sincerity and integrity — your friends, your family, your neighbors, your practice members, and even people you may only meet once in your life. Service changes the receiver and it changes the giver — YOU!

Chapter 5

"Some actors couldn't figure out how to withstand the constant rejection. They couldn't see the light at the end of the tunnel." – Harrison Ford

Law Five — Rejection

David K. Scheiner, D.C.

As children in this society you learn rejection relatively quickly. In fact, it occurs at birth for most people when you are birthed from the warm dark waters of your mothers womb and then immediately separated (the majority of babies), the cord is cut, and you are carried away by a masked stranger wearing blue latex gloves. You think to yourself, "I must either be in some horrible dream, in the wrong place, or both."

Most babies separated from their mothers at birth have the thoughts that they are not good enough, not wanted, and feel rejected. When you are finally returned to your mother you are confused. You're taken from the loving and nurturing environment you've known for 9 months and brought into a sterile atmosphere of cool rejection. This cements the tone in your subconscious of fear and fright.

Then when you are children and wandering, wondering, and using your imagination, you share these experiences with your teachers and parents, most of the time you are told that you have to draw within the lines and stay within the structures of the norm. The problem with this is that normal is broken. Most people lose their color, creativity and vision, where the world becomes black and white, fitting quite nicely within the walls of society; too scared to take risks because of their fear of rejection. You bring these fears with you throughout your lives in your relationships and in your work.

You must come to terms with this gathering of the fear of rejection and be willing to dance in the rain, be your unique self, remove the masks of your false selves, take the risks, follow the road less traveled, dare to be different, and most of all — live the life you love and love the life you live. Life is too short to care what others think and time is certainly not slowing down for you or anybody else.

The positive motivating force of rejection is necessary to experience so the beautiful unknown can be realized in your reality. Understand that it is not you who is being rejected or your thoughts and ideas. It is what you are projecting at that moment that is not fitting within the lines of the movie screen. You need to be willing to admit your strengths and powers. Say to yourself daily, "I am a powerful healer and I give myself permission to be empowered and strong." Continue with, "I have unique gifts to share with the world and I make a difference."

To truly be the person you came here to be you must be willing to develop the courage to stand at the edge of the cliff and take the leap, knowing that the winds of support and universal love will carry you effortlessly through the ether, delivering you at the doorsteps of your creatively unique, capable, and authentic self.

Brad Glowaki, D.C.

Because we have the perfect message, we get to be imperfect in the process of delivering it.

You are all going to make mistakes so get them out of the way. Do not be afraid to fail fast and fail forward. If the end result isn't what you were looking for, but you paid attention through the process, you've still gained at the end of the day.

The 8 Laws of Chiropractic Success

Once you figure out the recipe and the routine necessary to get the dynamite results, just rinse and repeat.

I'll end by saying, if you really make it about the patients and their needs, you cannot get rejected in the process. Rejection really comes down to ego and that is something you need to leave at the door.

Billy DeMoss, D.C.

If there's anyone who is an expert on rejection it would be me. I'm constantly pushing against the machine and pushing back on dogma. When you do that, you're going to get a lot of blowback. Rejection doesn't affect me like it did when I was looking to be accepted in my youth. As I slowly moved towards the light and my internal sight became strengthened, I began to stand for something. I became much more fulfilled, driven, and determined. I remember going to D.E. and listening to Dr. Sid say, "Stand for something or fall for everything," which I carry with me to this day.

I know that the movers and shakers you find on this journey have developed a rejection-proof vest of armor. To them, rejection is small and not something that will get in the way of sharing their message with the masses. These are the people you can really speak to and align with philosophically.

Allow rejection to be something you learn to love and embrace. Love your haters and if you don't have any then you're playing way too small.

Rejection is a badge of honor you should wear proudly. Realize there are always those who are in denial or so self-conscious that they have to take their insecurities out on you. Being a chiropractic warrior, you have set the stage for constant rejection. Continue to go against the grain of what's considered the norm of society and push against it. You will experience blowback but at the end of the day, like me, you'll wear your rejection badge of honor with pride.

The 8 Laws of Chiropractic Success

Amanda and Jeremy Hess, D.C.'s

I vividly remember one of my early mentors saying, "If you're not getting rejected a hundred times a day, you're doing something wrong." Rejection is normal and expected for those who go against the norm, the "sheeple" and the "machine."

Call it what you like, chiropractic and its principles of ADIO are counter-culture and will find the chiropractor, and anyone representing chiropractic, in a continual state of rejection. This is especially so for those of you whose hearts are about serving the people of your community in a big way and with multiple aspects of outreach. The fear of rejection has haunted many entrepreneurs, disruptors, and others who set out to chart a new course...the way us chiropractors do.

The only way to handle the fear of rejection is to start walking head-on into your fear and hit it hard. Start building "thick skin" by sharpening your chiropractic tongue and fighting the "battles within your mind." Once you gain momentum; face the fear, and start believing without a shadow of a doubt that God destined you to do what you're doing. The rejection may still come at times, but you will rarely get knocked down. Your recovery times will shrink to almost zero.

The chiropractors with the most robust practices are the ones who have used rejection in their favor and made it part of their headwind. Their messages of truth, conviction, and boldness keep them in the race of life, pressing on until the very end.

∞

Jason Deitch, D.C.

Rejection is one of those interesting concepts. By definition it means that someone refuses to accept your proposal or idea. However, the question you have to ask is "What if I stay persistent?"

Rejection is a feeling that kills practices and prevents people from discovering their story. It's a feeling to be aware of on your journey towards success.

You have to develop an awareness about how rejection

The 8 Laws of Chiropractic Success

influences what you do or do not do. You have to develop an internal force field, so to speak, so you do not take rejection personally. It's not personal at all. People reject your proposals and ideas most often because they are not "yet" in a position to say yes. It doesn't mean that they are rejecting you, it means they are not ready to say yes on your time table.

It is useful to remember that people say yes when they are ready to buy from you and not necessarily when you are ready to sell to them. You must remember that perhaps they'll say yes, next week, next month, next year, and under different circumstances but for today it might be a no. That's ok. In fact, it usually takes one-hundred no's before the first yes comes. And when the first one arrives, that opens the gates for the following ones to begin rolling in.

Yes, it's true, there are people with very fixed mindsets that may never accept your proposal or idea. However, the majority of rejection is due to timing and being aware of the social implications that impacts a person from accepting your idea. What impact would saying yes have on their social environment? Would their friends, family, or social circles criticize them if they said yes to you? Would they feel shame if they listened to your advice instead of their 'trusted' medical doctors' advice?

Listening for and looking at the reasons why someone may not say yes to you in the moment is essential to your ability to remain bold, communicate freely, and stay persistent and consistent with sharing your message and being of service to others.

∞

Claudia Anrig, D.C.

Get used to rejection. There are different stages in your life where you experienced rejection. When you didn't get picked for the team in elementary school — that was rejection. Get over it. The first time you asked somebody out for a date and was told "no" — that was rejection. Get over it.

Life goes on with or without those rejections. Get over

The 8 Laws of Chiropractic Success

rejection. Some people spend years on the psychologist's couch trying to get past the pain of rejection, but I'm telling you right now that everybody gets rejected.

When you want to move over to the left lane and the other cars won't let you in, are you going to get upset about that rejection? Think of rejection as another opportunity to do things differently. It's just another chance to help build character.

D.D. Humber, D.C.

When I first started in practice in the 1950's, rejection was faced by every Chiropractor. We were constantly bombarded by Medical Doctors and by every facet of the media who said that Chiropractic was unscientific, dangerous, based on a false premise, and those who practiced this profession were quacks, charlatans, and cultists.

> **Remember in health care today, it is Chiropractic first, medicine second, and surgery last.**

How would you like to face that type of opposition today? Well, it was not easy as many of our early pioneers in Chiropractic spent time in jail having been arrested for practicing medicine without a license. Dr. Herbert Ross Reaver carried the mantle of being the most jailed of all D.C.'s. He was incarcerated thirteen different times.

There may be D.C.'s today who feel that they are not accepted as well as they would like to be, but believe you me, acceptance of Chiropractic today is a thousand times better than what it was just a generation ago. If you are one that feels rejected, remember in health care today, it is Chiropractic first, medicine second, and surgery last.

Now, D.C. students and practicing Chiropractors alike, hold your head high. Face whatever rejection you must! Put the pedal to the metal, full steam ahead. Always remember — suffering humanity needs you and needs Chiropractic!

The 8 Laws of Chiropractic Success

Chuck Ribley, D.C.

Being a chiropractor, rejection is not part of my vocabulary. What I choose to do is to allow people to make informed choices. People either want what I have to offer or not. I do not make choices for other people. As a doctor I am the teacher, not the controller.

My mindset is that the innate understanding of ADIO is a principle that is forever unfolding in the hearts and minds of all people.

∞

Gerard Clum, D.C.

Rejection is about ego and the idea that whenever you do anything there's a service to be had. If it's your own ego you need to have served in the exchange and the exchange goes badly, you have a bad moment. But, if it's the well-being of your patient or the other person that you're trying to serve, then you do your best and if you're rejected, you can accept it *because* you did your best.

I remember walking with my son one Christmas when he was still a teenager and we passed a homeless guy on the street. When I slipped him a $20 bill, my son was aghast and asked, "Don't you know that he's just going to go buy beer or liquor with that?" I said, "I don't care, that's his choice. My choice was to make the gift and if he chooses to ruin his life with the gift or if he chooses whatever he needs at that moment, however irrational it may be to me, that's his choice."

If you involve yourself in what people do with what you put forward, it becomes personal and a reflection of you. It's no longer about what you've put forward but it's about them rejecting *you*. Reject my ideas, reject me is the way people look at things and when you look at it that way everything becomes personalized, which is where all of the hurt and fear comes from.

Rejection is everywhere. Rejection of the idea that may be put forward becomes painful only when it's personalized.

∞

The 8 Laws of Chiropractic Success

Donny Epstein, D.C.

Rejection is an interpretation of energy inefficiency in an interaction between individuals. What is being rejected usually is the energy state and consciousness that is impacting the field between you and that person who you are relating to. We are "punished" or "rewarded" by our energy efficiency in these interactions. When we drop the energy expression in the field (or don't effectively raise the coherent energy utilization) we and those we focus our attention on experience dis-ease, pain, or fear.

Raise the standard for expression of the conscious and effective use of our "personal" interactive energy in the field, and rejection is no longer relevant as it no longer exists. One's success in practice or in any business or endeavor is proportionate to one's willingness to risk rejection or confrontation.

Rejection is a reflection of the energy between people. The "rejector" is responding to the less than ecological use of energy by the person being rejected.

As an agent of healing, rejection is a calling for you to be more conscious and congruent in your use of energy and intelligence when interacting with the individual.

You must disappear, so to speak, and serve that individual's innate nature. Remember, there is no "I" in "We."

Ross McDonald and Rebecca Vickery, D.C.'s

Rejection is a tough yet powerful emotion to deal with as a chiropractor. For us, we generally believe that everyone can benefit from chiropractic. However, not everyone wants what we have to offer so it serves no purpose to take it personally. Sometimes we have to accept the decision and move on with the "SW" mantra — "Some will, some won't, so what, someone's waiting."

If we can learn to harness rejection, and perhaps more pertinently, the fear of rejection, this can lead to success in our chiropractic lives. Being fearful of rejection leads to inaction, stagnation, and certain failure.

The 8 Laws of Chiropractic Success

Rejection teaches us many things, one of which is patience. Harnessed properly, it teaches us to re-evaluate ourselves, our goals, and perhaps to change course and explore different paths in our journey, which otherwise wouldn't have been considered. Fundamentally, dealing positively with rejection creates opportunities for change and for personal and professional growth.

John Demartini, D.C.

Rejection lets you know that you are not communicating in accordance with the other person's values. That's inevitable at times, since you can't correctly determine everyone's values every single time. It's even harder if you're speaking before a group of people, since no statement you make will mesh with all their differing value systems. That's why rejection is part of the game.

If you aren't occasionally crucified, you probably aren't "on purpose." That, too, is part of the game. Any time you offer an original or novel idea, you're automatically going to get ridiculed and encounter violent opposition until that idea becomes a self-evident fact. You just have to endure the journey and stay the course with patience until whatever you do has been accepted and is seen in its true light.

Gilles LaMarche, D.C.

Rejection can serve as a detractor and disruptor for some people. For others, rejection is jet fuel to serve at an even higher level. If you never get rejected, you are not challenging the status quo. I remember being shy and fearful of sharing the chiropractic story until a mentor said, "What gives you the right to know a truth and not share it?" After asking his question multiple times while forcefully poking me in the chest with his index finger, I finally answered: "Nothing." He said, "That's right young man, nothing gives you the right to know a truth and not share it."

In that moment, I committed to doing whatever it took to

develop my communication skills. I did not focus on eliminating my shyness, I focused on developing my ability to communicate with power, passion, and certainty.

I adopted the position that some people might not want to hear what I had to say. I knew that some would and I would focus on them. Now, I'd never take rejection by others as an insult but rather as fuel to continue and say the powerful word "NEXT."

With a strong vision and purpose, you can face rejection and move on too. I know you can, no matter where you are at in your life.

Reggie Gold, D.C.

Well, chiropractors should feel rejected because of the way they promote and advertise chiropractic, which does not make any sense whatsoever. Why on earth would you want to be a straight chiropractor if your intention is to get rid of symptoms even though there are other ways of getting rid of symptoms besides chiropractic?

In fact, many symptoms are not caused by subluxation in the first place. Therefore, the straight chiropractor stands less chance of being successful than the mixer. The mixer can offer not only the adjustment, but physical therapy, which sometimes gets rid of symptoms; nutrition, which sometimes gets rid of symptoms; acupuncture, which sometimes gets rid of symptoms. They have lots of tools that the straight chiropractor doesn't have. If your intention is to get sick people well, you are much better off using other things as well as chiropractic.

Janice Hughes, D.C.

I love to share with clients that the faster and more often we get rejected, the more we learn to just get over it! Approval and/or rejection are quite simply over-rated. What do they have to do with your vision and mission? NOTHING.

I have learned in life that 50% of the people will love what

The 8 Laws of Chiropractic Success

you say and do, and 50% will hate it. No matter what you say and do! So ultimately the success principle is to focus on what is true for you and not others. By focusing on your vision and mission you will have some people that support and buy into it and others that reject it. If you can get into a place of understanding that your reactions to rejection are based on emotions, you can acknowledge it and quite simply move on.

In our Chiropractic lives, when you get stuck at the junction of rejection, you aren't effectively nor quickly able to move towards those that you can help and serve. In essence, the faster you get to a NO and don't react with emotion, the more quickly you get to the YES.

∞

Daniel & Richelle Knowles, D.C.'s

Some people are going to reject you simply because you shine too bright for them. That's okay. Keep shining.

I've mentioned to audiences around the world that as a chiropractor, you have chiropractic goggles on and see the world differently than others. Seeing the world this way, you're telling them it's round when they think it's flat. This sets the stage for a lot of rejection and ridicule. Rejection becomes your crucible, as it helps you grow and refine your communication. Keep telling the chiropractic story. It's your moral and ethical obligation to change lives for the better and in some cases save them.

The people you come in contact with are mostly on the road towards ill health. That will not change unless they have their trajectories of vision and mindset shifted. This important shift must occur for them and for their entire family regarding their health.

You have to have a vision bigger than rejection and realize that there's 7.8 billion people on the planet. Everyone deserves and needs chiropractic care. You can't take care of all of them, yet your vision ought to include them all. There will always be people that don't want what you have to offer but don't allow their rejection to get you down. It's your duty to sidestep the "No's" in order to find those willing to say "Yes." Stay the course.

The 8 Laws of Chiropractic Success

Thom Gelardi, D.C.

To be successful in any endeavor, you have to learn to face rejection. A famous salesmanship guru wrote that selling begins after the customer says "no." I kept on my desk at the college a card that said, "After the final no comes a yes and on that yes the future of the world depends."

The worst thing we can do is run away, physically or through the consumption of alcohol or drugs, from situations that are difficult for us. We grow by facing challenges. If rejection or some other situation is difficult for you, have a conversation with yourself as to what you'll do to overcome this aversion or fear. When you sincerely tell yourself that you'll face all of life's difficult situations, visiting the sick, visitations before funerals, public speaking opportunities, small talk at social gatherings, giving testimony in court, you're more than half-cured.

Know that the majority of people live fear-filled lives. They would rather follow the crowd that's filled with lost people following the crowd than think for themselves. Rather than thinking about being rejected, think about how you can better explain to the poor soul who rejected you or your idea. Remember also, don't take rejection personally. You're selling an idea and every salesperson knows that rejection is part of the selling game. Know when to stop wasting time trying to sell one prospect and move on to the next. The more doors one knocks upon, the more sales one makes.

Patrick Gentempo, D.C.

The issue of rejection is very significant in the chiropractic culture. Many chiropractors don't succeed because they have a fear of rejection, which prevents them from taking actions they should take.

Remember that, "All growth lives outside of the comfort zone." For many people, getting rejected is way outside their comfort zone and they don't want to put themselves in the position where somebody might reject what they're offering.

The 8 Laws of Chiropractic Success

For example, a chiropractor told me he was shopping and saw a woman in the drug aisle with her five-year-old girl, who had a cold. The mom was looking at the various labels on the drugs trying to determine which she would give to her child. The doctor wanted to approach her and ask her if she ever considered chiropractic care for her daughter or something to that effect. He managed to walk up to her but his fear of rejection stopped him from saying anything. He was unable to move outside his comfort zone and speak to the woman.

I told him the reason he didn't talk to her was because he made it about him. What every chiropractor has to understand is that this is not about you. It's about the people you're trying to help. In this doctor's case, the encounter wasn't about him; it was about the little girl. If his focus and attention had been on her instead of on his own fears, he would have opened his mouth.

You lose your fear of rejection when you stop being self-centered and focus on the people you want to serve. When you take yourself out of the equation, rejection is no longer an issue.

∞

Liam Schubel, D.C.

Your ability to achieve success in chiropractic will most likely be directly proportional to the level of fear you have of being rejected. Every offer for chiropractic care that you make opens an opportunity to grow your practice. Those who fear rejection in chiropractic generally take that rejection personally. You must remember that when people reject your offer of chiropractic care, they are not rejecting you. They are merely rejecting your offer. It is not personal.

The fact that some will reject your offer of chiropractic does not make chiropractic any less valuable. Chiropractic is a way to optimize one's life expression on this planet. What is that worth? Much of its worth depends on what people value. To some it is a more productive work environment, to some it is a better quality of life, and to others it will mean a life of less medication, less injections, and less surgeries.

The 8 Laws of Chiropractic Success

Imagine if you had an unlimited supply of gold bars. Your job in life was to hand those gold bars out to help people live better lives. What would happen to you if you offered a gold bar to someone and they rejected your offer? Would you think you are a bad person because they rejected your gold bars? Of course not! You would more than likely feel sorry for that person for not taking advantage of your generous offer.

> **I feel sorry for the person who rejected the offer. Now they have to live a life of greater fear and limitations.**

That is how I view rejection in chiropractic. I don't feel bad about myself. I feel sorry for the person who rejected the offer. Now they have to live a life of greater fear and limitations. Rejection doesn't make me feel bad about myself. It instead motivates me to improve my message so that I can help more people. I know that right around the corner is another yes and another opportunity to grow. Many times the universe tests whether you truly want the success you say you want in the world. Rejection for me is the universe saying, "Show me how bad you want it." Keep moving and call out, "Next!"

Sharon Gorman, D.C.

I have a friend who used to sell magazine subscriptions over the phone. He actually managed what they call a "boiler room," and he did much of the hiring. When he hired people he didn't look for the ones that had much success or acceptance in their life. He would hire people who had dealt with rejection. He knew that the people they called would reject them nine times out of ten but they wouldn't give up.

In the chiropractic world, one of the most effective ways to bring new patients into a practice is spinal screenings. This especially holds true in a new practice where there is not a large patient base to pull referrals from. When I hire someone to do screenings with me, I warn them that over 90% of the people who come to our booth will reject them. By telling them that, they aren't as disappointed when people don't oblige on-site. Don't allow rejection to stop you from telling people your truth and the truth of what chiropractic can do for them and their families.

My dad used to like to go on gambling trips that were paid for by the casinos. One time he was winning a lot of money and the pit boss was talking to my mom and my mom asked him, "Do you get mad when someone is winning and you know the casino is paying so much for them to be here?" He said, "No, the whole idea of the free trips is so that the casino gets "action." The casino knows that for every dollar played, a small percentage of that money will be theirs and therefore it doesn't matter if he wins or loses. It's always a numbers game.

I often think about that scenario with regards to the rejection that we endure in practice. If every patient I explained chiropractic to became a lifelong patient I would have stopped accepting new patients years ago because the administration of that many visits would be beyond what we could handle.

Kenny Rogers eloquently sings, "You have to know when to hold up, know when to fold up, know when to walk away, and know when to run."

∞

Jim Dubel, D.C.

I don't feel bad when someone has a pre-determined misconception about Chiropractic. It is inevitable that not every person will understand or comprehend the incredible value of a Chiropractic adjustment.

It's as simple as this, I share Chiropractic and my understanding of it with anyone that will listen. If someone chooses not to, I can't waste time arguing with them. I need to move on to the next person that might listen. It only takes one person at a time to understand our philosophy of Life.

The 8 Laws of Chiropractic Success

CJ Mertz, D.C.

Rejection goes back to the notion of "fail forward fast." The only person who can create rejection in your life is you. Recognizing that people really aren't rejecting you is a real breakthrough.

I love the story about the Hall-of-Fame baseball player who played ten to fifteen years in the Major Leagues and had a batting average of .300, which was good enough to make him one of the all-time best. A batting average of .300 means he failed to get a hit seven out of every ten times at bat, yet he was one of the greatest batters who ever lived. If he focused on the seven "failures" and took every pop-up, ground out, or strike out as a rejection, he would never have gotten the three hits out of ten that made him great.

No one has ever been perfect, so even thinking about being perfect is ridiculous. Fortunately, you don't have to be perfect in order to be great. Just make sure you keep your heart pure, your focus on right things, and never, ever take *anything* personally.

Larry Markson, D.C.

Fear of rejection is one of the biggest fears chiropractors have. Most feel their profession doesn't get enough respect and that people won't follow their recommendations. They think if they don't reduce a patient's visit frequency or waive the co-insurance fee, that person will leave. They feel rejected by the patient, so they lower their expectations of the patient's responsibilities just to get them to remain as patients.

Because I don't have that fear, I see volumes and volumes of people. Nationwide, the patient visit average (PVA) is around twenty or less but among my clients, the PVA is in the forties. The doctors I coach don't fear rejection; they tell their patients the truth and their patients get to accept, reject, or neutralize what they say. Patients have the right not to follow recommendations but when that happens, we don't feel rejected. I'm the doctor, they're the patients, and we both have responsibilities.

The 8 Laws of Chiropractic Success

Jeanne Ohm, D.C.

We plant seeds and try to have people come in to see us. We let them know that we'll be here when they're ready. They may get it — or they may not. If we feel rejected because of somebody else's choice or perspective, we're involving ourselves in something that has nothing to do with us.

The late Dr. Joe Flesia used to tell a great story related to this. You're a guest in a house and you wake up to find it's on fire. You run down the hall, knocking on the doors to all the rooms and telling them the house is on fire. Some people don't understand what you're talking about and no matter what you say, they roll over and simply go back to sleep. Do you stand there and attempt to explain and convince them or do you move on to the next room — to the person who may "get it" and want to be saved?

It's the same thing in your practice. Just keep moving on. Ask yourself if you explained things correctly and if the patient understood what you said. Look at the possibility that you were too abrasive, pushy, or didn't make your message clear enough. Look people in the eyes, go soul-to-soul, and allow your heart to dictate the conversation. If they get it and you resonate, that's wonderful. If they don't, you don't want them in your practice because they're going to cause trouble. Simply say, "Thank you Universe for letting me know that and let me move on."

Joe Strauss, D.C.

Rejection is something I really struggled with over the years and I suppose most people go through the same thing to some degree since nobody likes to be rejected.

Yet, I came to realize that it doesn't make sense to get upset or feel rejected just because someone doesn't come back to my office for a second visit or decides not to become a patient. My role is to give chiropractic care, share the philosophy, and spread the Big Idea to everybody in my community.

If people come in and listen to my message, they've allowed

The 8 Laws of Chiropractic Success

me to do what I need to do. Whether they accept it or not is not my responsibility. My responsibility is to make the chiropractic message as clear, concise, and desirable as I possibly can. What happens after that is not up to me. It's not my job or role to persuade people. I give them the information and let them make their own decisions.

Once I understood that, I no longer had to worry about rejection. I knew that if people didn't come back, it was because they just weren't ready for it.

Lou Corleto, D.C.

If you think you're not going to experience rejection, you should never have become a chiropractor. Rejection is inherent in chiropractic because of the stigma attached to the profession and the preconceived notions about what we do.

The trick is to not take it personally because it is *not about you.* Instead, try to learn from the experience (and this goes for all the rejections you experience in life, not just in chiropractic). If you feel someone is rejecting your chiropractic teaching, don't take it as a personal rejection but think about how you might improve the articulation of the message you're delivering.

Early in my career, I would feel horrible much of the time because I took people's reactions as personal rejections. One of the countless gifts I received from my teacher, Dr. Pasquale Cerasoli, is the lesson that chiropractic is for everybody but not everybody is for chiropractic.

You know that everyone can benefit from getting adjusted and when others choose not to do so, you can either feel rejected and judge them as ridiculous for not "getting it," OR, you can trust yourself and know that you did your best in that moment and then move on.

If people think you're a bit crazy for sharing the chiropractic concept, they're simply giving you free rein to go with that and be who you are. Take the gift — and go for it!

The 8 Laws of Chiropractic Success

Armand Rossi, D.C.

You'll hear a lot of negative things about rejection, but the fear of rejection almost singlehandedly made me successful. I was so afraid I would be rejected by my family and all the other people who expected me to do well, that success became an important goal.

Yet, for most doctors, fear of rejection isn't a motivating force. Instead, they're so afraid of being rejected they freeze up. They won't go out of the office and look for new patients or talk to new people or tell the truth about chiropractic because they're afraid of rejection. One of the things Dr. Jim Sigafoose taught me was to make it a game and see how many times I could be rejected in a single day. That helped a lot.

Christopher Kent, D.C.

It's not the rejection itself but the fear of the rejection that prevents individuals from doing what they know is right. You need to realize that if you don't do something, you are already rejected. As a friend of mine used to say, "If you don't ask the question, the answer is always no." Do you want certain rejection or do you want possible rejection? So do it!

Tedd Koren, D.C.

I remember being rejected a lot by girls when I was younger. Did I stop looking? Of course not! I just kept on looking for the next one. Rejection can either be a stumbling block or a stepping stone for you. It's really your choice.

When I was trying to get on radio and TV in the Philadelphia area, I made call after call but got rejected each time. It didn't stop me then either — I just learned from the experience and finally figured out how to deal with media people. When I made it a learning experience instead of a personal rejection, I ended up on every one of those stations. After one of the first talk shows I was on, I had eighty-three new patients that week. Not bad. Those kinds of numbers continued, dropped a bit, and went on that way for many weeks.

Because of the initial rejections, I learned how to do it right. I knew I had a tremendously important message to deliver that was more important than the personal implications of being rejected. I actually wrote a book from the experience called, "How to Get on Radio and TV."

Ever since then, I've learned to use rejection as a teaching and motivating tool. When I was attacked by the federal government, it didn't bring me down. Instead, it actually helped me create other products for our patient education line.

Terry A. Rondberg, D.C.

Like so many adversities in life, rejection is a negative emotion which is a direct result of feeling inferior. As a chiropractor, I faced rejection almost from day one. My own relatives rejected my professional choice! One of my wife's relatives actually reacted by flailing her hands in the air, gesturing me away with a vehement cry of, "Oh no, a chiropractor! Stay away from me." I told her I really had no desire to go near anyone with that attitude.

In reality... rejections can be great spiritual opportunities to grow.

When we experience this type of rejection, it's sometimes hard to maintain a healthy self-esteem. But if you believe strongly in the benefits of chiropractic and know that you're giving a valued service, the pride you feel in yourself and your profession will overcome that type of reaction.

You just have to realize that rejection is part of the game. Speak up and be proud of what you do. You may face rejection but don't let it stop you or affect you negatively. You have the choice. It can only hurt you if you choose to allow it to. In reality, such rejections can be great spiritual opportunities to grow.

The 8 Laws of Chiropractic Success

Jessica Harden, D.C.

I have often heard it said that, "If you are not being rejected you are doing something wrong." What is it that you are doing wrong? Perhaps the best explanation comes from William Burnbach, the legend of the advertising industry. He said, "If you stand for something, you will always find some people for you and some against you. If you stand for nothing, you will find nobody against you and nobody for you."

We must take a stand in what we believe in. As chiropractors, we have a unique science, philosophy, and art to approach health. Simply representing these ideas with a D.C. degree would attract rejection. One must be comfortable with rejection and have the courage to tell others "The Story" of chiropractic.

If you are noticing very little rejection on your journey to success, you are either playing it safe or hiding.

Teri and Stu Warner, D.C.'s

Michael Jordan, considered one of the greatest basketball players of all time, openly admits to failing more than most. He has been quoted as saying, "I lost almost three hundred games (that's more games than many NBA players have court time in), missed over nine thousand shots (again more shots than an average NBA player ever takes), and twenty-six times I was given the ball to take the game winning shot and MISSED." Ironically, Jordan says the reason he has succeeded boils down to his constant failure. He did not allow failure to equal his defeat. He used it as motivation for success and as stepping stones towards victory.

Setbacks are inevitable and it is our perception of that 'failure' which means the difference between achieving success or not. A hall of fame baseball player, the best of the best, strikes out seven out of ten times at bat. Should he be disappointed that he failed 70% of the time? What would happen if we quit because we were rejected by seven out of ten patients?

The first big lesson for you to learn in practice is, "No doesn't

The 8 Laws of Chiropractic Success

mean No, it just means, Not Yet." When you hear the word "No," never take it personally. Get used to rejection, it's what happens in practice and in life, every day. Many patients don't follow direction, some will discontinue care (even after getting miracle results), but don't interpret this rejection as failure. Redefine the rejection and turn it into something positive that will drive and inspire you.

Redefine the rejection and turn it into something positive that will drive you and your message...

If opportunity doesn't knock, build a new door on your failure and use it as a stepping stone. Close the old door to the past and don't let it haunt you. Learn from your mistakes, don't dwell on them, don't let them steal your passion, and don't let them sabotage your success. Redefine the rejection and turn it into something positive that will drive you and your message to serve more patients and achieve massive success.

∞

Neil Cohen, D.C.

How you handle rejection is the difference between success and lack of success. Although rejection is often perceived as personal, it should never be taken personally! Not everyone wants everything you have to offer all of the time.

When your beloved Chiropractic is rejected or a patient does not return to your office, emotion should be absent from your mind. Many of you rarely apprehend this concept because of your attachments to money, ego, recognition, the outcome, and here's the really big one...FEAR!

What are you afraid of? Understand that rejection builds your character. Do not lose heart! Deliver the goods, whether they be the adjustment or the message and move on to the next blessed soul you are to touch with those magnificent hands. Students and doctors, be specific, become a master, and Illegitimi non carborundum — "Don't let the bastards grind you down."

Paul Reed, D.C.

Rejection is an area of frustration for many chiropractors that I work with. The unfortunate thing is that they have not embraced it. I believe it is a really good thing and part of our circle of chiropractic life. You chiropractors were placed here to be warriors of truth, guardians of health, and angels of life; forging your way against the raging seas.

I like to reference the Rhino when discussing rejection with chiropractors. Rhinos possess a thick resilient skin that protects them as they crash through the rough terrains. I believe that each one of you must travel the highways and bi-ways, sharing the chiropractic health and healing principles to all who will and will not listen. This gives you the opportunity to hone your communication skills and develop your "Rhino Skin." This will make you stronger in practice when you give your patients recommendations that they are not expecting to hear. This strength, passion, and conviction will enable you to stay true to your principles, not having you take the road *more* traveled, at this time of rejection.

After years of practice, I now understand why so much of the population rejects us. I offer you these time-tested and proven tools in order for you to move the chiropractic needle into its successful position in society.

Steve Judson, D.C.

There is no such thing as rejection; just temporary confusion in value not understood. When your intention is right you should never give up on your vision or your mission of serving the masses.

When walking the halls as a student at Life University, I'd read a statement up high on the wall, "Persistence Is Omnipotent." No one is rejecting you. They may be rejecting an idea or offer — not you.

Persist until they can see what is needed in order to feel the truth of our glorious Principle. There is not one soul who does

The 8 Laws of Chiropractic Success

not need what you have in your hands and within your hearts. They will accept it when they are ready for the change that we already see in them.

Tim Young, D.C.

Rejection is an interesting concept. I, like many of you, have struggled with rejection or the fear of it. I will make this as easy as I can. Rejection is not you responsibility. Acceptance is not your responsibility. The only responsibility that you have to your patients, your family, or to the world, is to tell the truth as you know it and deliver on that truth time and time again.

If others choose to accept your truth or not, this too, is not you responsibility. Deliver your truth and let the universe take care of the rest. The sooner you grasp this concept the faster success will come.

Frederick A. Schofield, D.C.

In every practice there's an aspect of rejection. There are many voices in practice. The internal dialogue of patients is different than the internal dialogue of the doctor, they speak a different language. Patients have different voices in their head: the Voice of Rejection, the Voice of Fear, the Voice of Anxiety, the Voice of Hostility, and the Voice of Apprehension; all part of the Voice of Threat. So, the Doctor has to minimize the Voice of Threat by what's known as Situational Confrontation.

Rejection comes from your last experience. The key to neutralize rejection is to agree with love and compassion to those voices that feel threatened. Patient: "Dr. I don't want to come here for the rest of my life!" Doctor: "Relax, I agree with you, you are absolutely right." And in that agreement you neutralize the Voice of Rejection. Remember, before every YES is a No.

Be Still and Sow and SO IT IS!!!

Cathy Wendland-Colby, D.C.

Some will. Some won't. So what. Who's next. Get that through your head.

If you plan to have an impact on your community, you better have thick skin. Some people will absolutely love you, your office, your brand of Chiropractic, and some won't. It's just a fact of life, so you accept it and move on. You can't please everyone, so why kill yourself bending over backwards for the few who don't want what you have? You'll risk missing the opportunity to help someone who truly needs and values your care. Devote your time in service to those who resonate with you and you will find more joy and peace in your practice and in your life.

Honestly, rejection is part of the cycle of things. When you ask for anything in life, sometimes the answer is yes and other times it will be no. It's OK. So what. Move on. Who's next?

Guy Riekeman, D.C.

My friend, bestselling author Barbara DeAngelis, has written often about the relationship between anger, hurt, fear, and rejection.

Anger always stems from some hurt, and hurt always comes from fear. If you have no fear, you can't be hurt. Rejection is some result of fear and hurt you have in your life.

For instance, someone could say to me, "You're the ugliest guy I've ever met in my life." If I have a strong image of myself, such a statement wouldn't hurt me or be interpreted as rejection. But if I'm insecure about my looks, I'd feel rejection. I'd feel hurt, and from that I'd ultimately feel anger.

You avoid a sense of rejection by stabilizing your internal resources regarding what you believe, what you know to be true, what you want to give to humanity, and what you're willing to take on in order to do that.

Brian Kelly, D.C.

When I first applied to Chiropractic College I wasn't accepted. I was finally accepted very late in the enrollment process after a student who had been accepted, declined the colleges offer. Since that initial rejection, I have served thousands of patients, run a Research Organization, been appointed President of two Chiropractic Colleges in two countries, and received numerous professional awards, in my first 26 years in chiropractic. Today, I speak to chiropractic audiences worldwide and coach chiropractors on how to achieve the practice and life of their dreams.

It is said that success leaves clues. It is possible that so-called rejection does as well.

I could have taken not being accepted into Chiropractic College as rejection, yet how would that have served me and others?

If you fail an exam as a student, are you a failure or are there valuable insights to be gained? Could you have studied harder? Could you have studied?! Could you have developed a greater understanding of the work? I used to wonder who is better off, the person who passes an examination at 51% or the one who fails at 49% and has to re-take the test.

It has been said there is no such thing as failure, only feedback. If a patient declines your care or stops your care, it may be about you and your office, or not about you at all. However, it may be about you if you are always running late, if you gossip about your patients, if you have an unorganized office with unfriendly hours, etc. In this context, the so called 'rejection' is great feedback.

What can you learn and how can you improve? You must always look for patterns and themes in your office and in your own life. It is said that success leaves clues. It is possible that so-called rejection does as well.

The 8 Laws of Chiropractic Success

Kevin Jackson and Selina Sigafoose-Jackson, D.C.'s

Rejection is a double edged sword in that it can allow you to grow by learning what makes people tick and what you can change about how you present things. Rejection can also allow you to become mentally tough. James Sigafoose, D.C. used to talk about being a member of the "rejection club" where getting rejected was like a badge of merit.

When you're telling people the chiropractic story not everyone is willing to accept it. But much like Babe Ruth, you have to strike out in order to hit some home runs. So never be afraid of rejection in chiropractic, especially if you are giving a solid explanation of what chiropractic is. Have reasonable fees and practice at a high level when locating and correcting vertebral subluxation. Rejection can ultimately make you a better chiropractor and person.

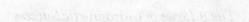

Chapter 6

"Love is the great miracle cure. Loving ourselves works miracles in our lives." – Louise L. Hay

Law Six — Love

David K. Scheiner, D.C.

First and foremost you must find the love for yourself before you can truly love, give, or receive with another. Love is the cornerstone of the universe and since the universe is energy, light, and eternal life, everything begins and ends here. Love is eternal and like the effects of the chiropractic adjustment, it has the potentiality to transform lives.

When we see ourselves and others for what we and they actually are (pure energy) then we can begin to truly live and be free. You came here to live a life you love and to live it powerfully. You must develop the confidence to know that you will live a powerful and loving life; being of great service to others. The ONLY way you will experience joy, love, and magic in your life is by having your chiropractic career be transformative for yourself and therefore those you serve. Work constantly with the clusters of fears you accumulate in life (rejection, betrayal, humiliation, abandonment, etc.) in order to not keep love at a distance.

In order to be a healing agent of change and transformation, the time of battling yourselves and others must close. The need to be perfect and the illusion of falling short can be gently placed aside. The need to control and struggle can be given up so you can easily make your way to the sacred unknown where true love resides. It is within this beautiful, sacred, and mystical unknown where we all come together and experience the resonant tone D.D. Palmer, D.C. spoke of long ago. Love manifests here and as we practice our healing craft, the healing of the people and planet shall occur — every time — through love.

Brad Glowaki, D.C.

Love is the most powerful emotion on planet Earth.

The more people have the opportunity to feel it through a non-invasive, non-drug, and non-surgical technique to their body, the more it allows them to express love at a higher level.

When people feel loved in a chiropractic practice, that practice never fails. Therefore, love *is* the secret ingredient, the essence of what we do, and what we need to provide, in order for success to be experienced by those we serve and ourselves.

Teri and Stu Warner, D.C.'s

There are many kinds of love. Love of God, love of self, love of Chiropractic... all of which play a pivotal role in personal and professional success. It is our experience that at the foundation of these types of love is an innate sense of love of self from which health, happiness, and success emanates and flourishes..

Design your practice to be 'love-centric.' Surround yourself with staff who love, value, and support you, and who love chiropractic. Purposefully exude a love for your patients regardless of their faults or flaws. See the perfection in others and connect with them on an innate level.

Love your patients and build them up, while connecting with them on an emotional level. Don't just be there to physically adjust them. Staying engaged and "in the zone," always giving the patient in front of you your undivided attention (whether that's a newborn, pediatric, adult, or elderly patient), will build long-term wellness care relationships fortified with trust.

The 8 Laws of Chiropractic Success

The longer we are in practice, the more in love we are with it, and the simpler it gets. We do our best to follow the guiding principle of the Lasting Purpose: To Give, To Do, To Love, To Serve — out of a sense of abundance with a burning desire to serve our community and our fellow man. The bible says, "Love your neighbor as yourself." Share this love and joy with your family of patients. The love will exude from within you, without you ever having to say a word. The rest is easy and will take care of itself.

Amanda and Jeremy Hess, D.C.'s

Love in the Chiropractic practice is best revealed by, "Doing unto others as you would have done unto yourself." Putting these words into action with yourself and your team is crucial for long-term stability and growth for any Chiropractic practice wanting continued success.

Living by this mantra, you care for your practice members the same way you care for your own family. You inherently show your team high-level sincerity and steadfastness in the process. You're continually creating an atmosphere of love and caring that penetrates your team. Now you've built a dynamic of uncommon loyalty, respect, and longevity with both your practice members and, even more importantly, your team members.

Don't allow your love to come across as insincere and exaggerated. Love is simply a process of repeated action on a daily basis of what you know to be right for your practice members regardless of the opinions of others.

Arno Burnier, D.C.

Love has been called the ingredient of universal synthesis. Every single book I've ever read about healing said that love was a crucial component. Whether people were healing through food, acupuncture, massage, bodywork, chiropractic, or surgery, love was an essential ingredient.

The 8 Laws of Chiropractic Success

It's also been the message in all the great spiritual and religious books throughout the ages. It's a perennial philosophy and understanding that love is the essence of life and Christ was a perfect example of love as the power to heal.

When people come to me with their compelling stories of suffering, my heart opens wide and something leaps out of me when I touch them. At such moments, far more happens than would have happened had the adjustment been delivered without my heart opening up with love.

Janice Hughes, D.C.

Love and passion are on the same spectrum, or simply a gradient of each other. Love isn't only about relationships in our life, it's about our relationship TO life!

We can all identify people with that 'something extra,' that vitality. They pour themselves whole heartedly into anything they are doing. Watch them parent (yes even in those challenging times), watch them meet new people, and listen to them talk about things they are interested in. These are the people that will share with you that even within the challenges, even with obstacles in their path, the more they embrace this life and learn...the more they grow.

We get one day at a time and one life to LIVE. By choosing to love it we bring passion and zest to all that we do. Bringing that energy to practice and to building your Chiropractic career enables you to move mountains and align the stars to harness your dreams.

John Demartini, D.C.

Love is the synthesis and synchronicity of complementary opposites and when you adjust a spine, you're bringing the complementary opposites into equilibrium. You are basically a love generator. I always think of chiropractic as an art, science, and philosophy of love.

Chuck Ribley, D.C.

Love is an attraction, a vibrational force, and an affinity of energies coming together. I know my energy of love goes out into the world and people who vibrationally are attracted to me will pass by many chiropractors and come to my office.

When I am in tune with my Innate I am in tune with my patients Innate and at that sacred time there in that space, you might say I become one with the bone and one with that patient. B.J. Palmer, D.C. called it adjusting with that something extra.

∞

Jessica Harden, D.C.

When unconditional, love is a powerful force that drives our actions and attitudes. Biblically, it is said that love can conquer all and if you live knowing unconditional love, you can attest to it!

There are never guarantees in life. Events can happen overnight that completely transform it. Endurance through these changes can be fueled by unconditional love. Love for yourself, love for your Maker, love for your family, profession, and business.

Some may ask how can you continuously channel unconditional love? Considering our imperfections, it's not always easy but with steady daily practice it can become easier. It starts with a conscious choice, the decision to filter actions and responses through unconditional love.

It takes daily prayer and meditation to continually make that decision every day coupled with finishing the day remembering the result and reward of those actions and thoughts. If you can find this unconditional love every day, you discover an unmatched anchor to keep you grounded on your path of success.

Neil Cohen, D.C.

For those of you that embrace the Chiropractic philosophy, love becomes a grander way of thinking. The life of a principled chiropractor transcends Chiropractic. You are innately compelled to walk differently, talk differently, act differently, and think differently. The way you order your life ought to continuously be from love. I can hear, at this moment, the powerful and gentle voice of Dr. Sid Williams saying "Let love be your master."

In Chiropractic terms, love ought to be considered a cumulative, constructive, survival value simply because it never fails. Accordingly, the New Testament upholds this great truth regarding love; declaring that love is patient, love is kind, love protects, love trusts, love hopes, and love perseveres. Additionally, the scripture declares that love does not dishonor others, it is not self-seeking, it is not easily angered, and it keeps no record of wrongs.

Love IS your first and greatest technique in your life and your practice. Students, your hearts are to remain open as you navigate your way into becoming an experienced and successful leader and practitioner in your communities. Wounds and battle scars will make you weary but they too build character as you keep your mind and heart unconditionally wide open.

Love is not just an emotion; it is a verb and an action word. Be active, responsive, and energetic with the love that you carry within you. Your love will never deplete as other commodities often do. When you generously and freely give your love away, dividends and increase will result, earning you more love and abundance than you had before. By being motivated in and through love, your rewards will be counted to you as glorious, yielding the fruit of a peaceful spirit and insurmountable joy.

Frederick A. Schofield, D.C.

Johann Wolfgang von Goethe stated, *"The moment one definitely commits oneself, then providence moves into. Whatever you think you can do, I'll believe you can do, begin it. Action has magic, power, and grace."*

Loving service is the first law of creating an infinity of trust and loyalty with your patients. The first aspect of love, in practice, is to thank the patient for choosing your office. We build strong relationships that create lifetime patients through passion and the love of what you do through the service we provide.

Dr. Jim Parker said, "Loving service, my first technique." The environment that you create empowers the unique and personalized experience with your patients. Love your patients thru:

1) Agreement
2) Acknowledgment
3) Thankfulness

LOVE IS IN THE FREQUENCY

Be Still and Sow and SO IT IS!!!

Guy Riekeman, D.C.

One of the principles in chiropractic is that for any given amount of matter there is one-hundred percent intelligence and it's always proportional to its needs. In our society we see everything as limited and finite resources. We see love that way as well. We see it like a pie: if I give a slice to one person, I have that much less to give to someone else.

When my first daughter was born I loved her one-hundred percent. When the second child was coming, I wondered how I'd be able to love her as much as I did my first, without taking anything away from the first. When the second one came, I found out I loved her one-hundred percent too, and it didn't take anything away from the first.

There's an unlimited amount of love in the universe and it's always proportional to its requirements. There's an unlimited amount of health in the universe and in your body, and it's always proportional to its requirements.

If you can't love what you do and can't love the people who are coming in (and not necessarily for who they are or what they do, but simply for the possibility of who they can become) your practice is just going to be a business to you.

That's why at Life University we spend time talking about Lasting Purpose, which is To Give, To Serve, To Love, and To Do out of a sense of abundance.

The 8 Laws of Chiropractic Success

Billy DeMoss, D.C.

Love is up there with the most important aspects of success. For you to be ultimately successful, you have to love what you do and truly love those you serve. For most, negativity and hate are automatic; it takes courage to be a beacon of light, love, and truth for your community.

In my daily life I make it a point to interact positively with the people I meet, whether it be the person who is helping me at the airport or someone who is coming in for their first adjustment. I want to receive it back, so that's what I give.

Most people around the globe never experience love, let alone a kind word or gentle touch. I suggest you join me in putting out as much love as possible to the entire world. Together we will turn the tide, where the hungry are fed, the neglected are attended to, and the unloved are embraced with the unfathomable beauty they so desire and deserve.

Claudia Anrig, D.C.

Chiropractic *is* love. Love of showing up every day, love of service, and love of adjusting a newborn baby. Nothing is more humbling to me than when parents bring me their first newborn and ask me to check and adjust their beloved. To me, that's the fullest expression of love — when parents actually present their child to me because they know I love them like a brother or sister, or just because they're human beings on the planet.

We're very blessed and we get to love people every day in our practices and be loved back. Not too many people can say that, so we're very fortunate.

Ross McDonald and Rebecca Vickery, D.C.'s

Love is a key component of success and fulfilment in chiropractic. We must have a passion for what we do as chiropractors, a desire to serve our communities and make positive change, and a reverence for the power of the human being to heal and repair when there is no longer interference in the nervous system.

Wayne Dyer stated, "Doing what you love is the cornerstone of having abundance in your life." It is an energy and a mindset which positively impacts the interaction we have with those we come into contact with.

∞

D.D. Humber, D.C.

"Loving *service, my first technique"* was taught by Dr. Jim Parker at his Parker Seminars. Dr. Sid Williams, my friend, colleague, mentor, and boss for more than a quarter century, greatly expanded this concept relating to Chiropractic practice. He and Dr. Nell also based their lives on this concept and encouraged others to do the same. It is known as the *Lasting Purpose Principle*: To love, to serve, to give, and to do. If you— as a Chiropractic student or a D.C.— will adopt this concept, this principle, as it were, it will go a long way in assuring your success.

The Scriptures teach that God is love. When one truly loves what they do and loves those they serve, it is impossible to fail. Learning to love others is so needed in this world today and we as Doctors of Chiropractic can and must lead the way!

∞

Paul Reed, D.C.

Love is one of our greatest commandments and is a cornerstone of every successful chiropractic practice. The more you pour out an expression of love and joy to your patients, the greater their healing experience is going to be in your practice.

Today's practice members come in with more stress, worry, dis-ease, and separation from their source than ever before. Combating these things with love expedites the healing process. People are touched, hugged, and loved so little today that it is an opportunity for us to fulfill one of the greatest commandments by just being who you are.

The 8 Laws of Chiropractic Success

I've intentionally made it a habit to speak love to the youth in our practice. I do this by addressing them with power words; calling them beautiful, gorgeous, good looking, rock star, amazing, etc. They too are missing the affection they had just a few years ago. Regularly speaking love over them helps to pay immediate dividends in their life and for generations to come.

Cathy Wendland-Colby, D.C.

Have you ever been the Jenny to someone's Forrest Gump? That type of unwavering, non-judgmental, and unconditional love? If you have, hopefully you handled it well and didn't crush the poor guy. But if you're like a lot of people who will come into your office, the last time they felt anything that even came close to that was back when they were in diapers and Mom was still oohing and ahhing over her newborn.

Let them see through you what an extraordinary life looks like...

How about exuberant joy? This is also missing in the lives of many of your prospective patients. I'm willing to bet that you know people who hit the snooze button on life a long time ago and are just sleepwalking around like a bunch of sheeple sitting in traffic, working in cubicles, and crashing out on the sofa for a few hours of mind numbing TV.

It's time we wake them up and shake them up. Let them see through you what an extraordinary life looks like, what abundant happiness feels like, how easy it is to make healthier choices, and experience the magic of sharing unconditional love. I'm not saying that you have to teach anyone anything other than ChiropracTIC. Just let them feel what it's like to be around people vibrating at a higher frequency in your office. Give, love, and serve out of your own abundance, with no expectation of anything in return, and with the absolute understanding that the universe always provides.

Gerard Clum, D.C.

If you don't love what you're doing, it becomes a mechanical thing. You might be economically successful or not, but love makes the thing joyful.

So many people think this is unique to chiropractic but if you had to have coronary bypass surgery, which of two equally skilled surgeons would you choose: the one who was thinking the procedure would pay the next month's mortgage, or the one who enjoyed performing surgery more than anything else in life?

It's the love of what you do, of the effect you can have, of the interaction with people, and the desire to help them that takes things to a different level. Competency be damned — if I have to have my chest cracked open, I want people who love what they're doing to do it. Love is the kind of variable that changes people's lives. We all recognize it when we see it and are aware when it's absent.

Liam Schubel, D.C.

In a world today that is filled with cold technology and automation, the chiropractic office is still a place where people can come to fill up on love. One of the biggest complaints that people have about the modern health care delivery system is its coldness. Practice members many times feel like numbers or "workloads" for the doctors' offices that they enter into. It's all about the insurance forms, paperwork, prescriptions, and test results.

One of the huge keys to success in business is obviously marketing. The unique selling proposition in your business is what sets you apart from others and helps to establish your value in the market. Sadly, in the health care field in general, love is absent. If you can provide an environment that has, at its fundamental core, a place where loving service is the norm then you will be unique. People won't remember so much the things you say to them but they will remember that you made them feel loved. They will refer their friends and family to you because they

The 8 Laws of Chiropractic Success

will know an experience in your office is a welcomed refresh from what they are accustomed to. They want to feel loved and they want results.

When I started to take care of Latino practice members in the USA, the importance and scarcity of love-based health care became brutally apparent. On the first office visit I would warmly welcome them to my practice and then ask how I could serve. Many would start to cry. At first I thot it was because they were in pain. "What's wrong?" I asked? The response was shocking. "You are the first doctor in this country that has treated me like a human being."

What a sad commentary on our health care system, but a huge opportunity for those of us that can serve our practice members with love in our hearts, words, and actions. We can truly be the change that we wish to see in the world. Love rules!

Steve Judson, D.C.

Love is blindness and has become the greatest secret in the world. When humanity lives clear and connected they WAKE UP! When they awaken, the love within rises to the top and Unlocks the Purpose for their life. As you love yourself, you are then able to love others. This takes work and effort. The more you love, the greater the expression of life becomes. Similarly, the more you fulfill your life purpose, the more love, gratitude, and peace you'll feel within. This is the essence of transforming lives; first your own and then others.

You must realize the gift you have to offer humanity as chiropractors. This gift is something everyone needs, yet they are unaware of it. It is their right to live a clear and connected life and your duty to spread the message far and wide.

Be relentless and rejection-proof spreading your message. Create a tsunami of love.

∞

Tim Young, D.C.

I believe love is the first foundation of any success. Not the kind of love you might first think. Dr. Parker would say that Loving service is our first technique. I agree, but in the case of being successful in chiropractic or in any business or relationship, you must first love yourself. If you don't love, trust, respect, admire, look up to, and believe in yourself, how can you possibly expect anyone else to?

Love of who you are is a daily exercise that should be practiced with as much focus and intention as anything else you do. The greater the love you have for who you are, the greater the clarity you will have for what you do and why you do it. This is where ultimate success starts and for many, stops before it starts.

Gilles LaMarche, D.C.

Have you ever asked yourself, "Is there a deeper and more real version of myself waiting for the right time to show up but for the most part, letting that person out seems just way too risky?" I know I have and I also know that I was fearful of being my real, genuine, and authentic self.

Then one day I realized that being real, genuine, and authentic without the need to impress, pretend, feel shame or fear was the only person I could be. It was then that I chose to start playing this game of life full-out. From that day forward I made the decision to show-up real, vulnerable, without judgement, and with my eyes and heart wide open. I chose to show-up in life as the kind loving soul that I was born to be. Just like you were born to be.

The power of unconditional love is immeasurable and love is the most powerful energy on the planet. After all, negative feelings toward others punish me on the spot, for I am a chained slave to anyone I dislike.

As chiropractic students and chiropractors, it is important that you discover and experience how unconditional love truly is the magic bullet of all healing — physical, mental, and spiritual.

The 8 Laws of Chiropractic Success

For some people you interact with, the unconditional love and respect you offer them might be the only time they feel what you are sharing.

You may want to rewrite the script of your life and taste the vulnerability of true love by allowing yourself to love others unconditionally. There is no force more powerful, no food more enriching, and certainly no drink more tasty or more quenching than unconditional love.

Jim Dubel, D.C.

Do I Love Chiropractic? You Bet I do! Do I Love patients that understand and receive care? Absolutely!

I go out of my way to accept and understand each patient in a loving way, knowing that every patient has different concerns and reasons to be under Chiropractic care. I personally try to extend unconditional love to them from my own abundance.

Jason Deitch, D.C.

Khalil Gibran, author of The Prophet, wrote, "Work is love made visible."

Love relates to everything, always. Love for yourself. Love for your craft. Love of being of service to others. Love for your work. Love of achievement. Love for making an impact. It was once said that, "The more you love something, the more it reveals its secrets to you."

Loving yourself, loving your work, loving the opportunity to share your gifts with as many people as possible is what drives all *successful* chiropractors.

Sharon Gorman, D.C.

I love that word, it makes me feel good. Aren't we all looking for love? Sometimes when I find myself looking for love it is because

I don't feel loved; usually because I'm not giving enough love away to others.

I think God is love. I experience God by experiencing the love of other people and by allowing people to love me. All of us that have loved, which is all of us, have been hurt by people who we love and who we let love us. We're all human beings and therefore bring our personality flaws along with us into our loving relationships. When we get hurt by the people we love, we retreat and protect ourselves, cutting off from being loved. In this place, it is virtually impossible to filter love so we shut down. This is one of the worst things we can bring on to ourselves.

Loving our pets is much safer and is the reason so many people bond with their animals more than they bond with and love people. I have this dog I really love and when I see her, I often bite my bottom lip with emotion. There's no doubt that she likes me but I feel so much love every time I look at her because of my *experience* loving her. I want you to get that "I feel love *when* I love." Maybe loving a dog is taking the easy road, but what the hell, go for it. Love is love and it's better to love and be loved than not to love at all.

I feel so much love for my patients. When I was in practice the first four years, I was seeing patients and running four individual practices. I got married and in a few years we started having kids. In four years we had four kids. People would tell me all the time that I was crazy and looking back they were probably right. At home, I loved my family and in the office I loved my staff and my patients. It is hard to feel anything but love when you are so busy loving and being loved. Love feels so good.

Daniel & Richelle Knowles, D.C.'s

Susan Barbara Apollon said, "When your heart is filled with the energy of love and deliberately focused on a person or place, there is an energetic shift and healing is expedited."

Love is the most basic human need and love is the vital key

to healing. Love all of your patients. Not just the ones that prepay. Not just the ones that make it to their appointments. Not just the ones that are good looking. Not just the ones that have fancy cars. Not just the ones that dress well. Love all of them.

Always see within your patients the inner champion imprisoned within them that hasn't expressed itself fully yet. We have a phrase in our office that states, "The worst ones are the best ones." My wife, Dr. Richelle, came up with that saying. The ones that we think are the "bad" new patients or the "challenging" ones often become the best ones. They've been living life at less than their optimal potential due to structural distortions. It's no wonder why they are difficult to deal with at the outset.

Create a community within your office and make it a place where people feel loved, wanted, and welcomed. Imagine your office as an oasis within a magical bubble that encapsulates a loving, giving, and serving environment. It is a place where they feel safe; a place where they can be vulnerable and heal. Let all of that come through in your touch, in your eyes, in your hug, in your posture, and in your communication with people. How people are treated makes a tremendous difference in their capacity to heal.

Rumi said, "Love is the bridge between you and everything." Therefore, love your practice members without limits while also allowing love to flow to you.

Jeanne Ohm, D.C.

Everyone who comes into your office is a body needing to love and be loved. That's their biggest need in life. Whatever their health issues or whatever else is going on with them, it's all about not feeling loved enough.

Let's make sure we treat all people (in and out of our offices) with love and respect. Let's not forget that we too are in need of love and never at any point are we higher or better than any of them. We may have, or be able to share, a different perspective on something but that doesn't make us better than anyone else.

Do the best you can and love yourself for that. If you're truly giving of yourself with love, it will light a spark in others and they will connect with it. Maybe they won't run into your office that day and commit to lifetime care, but you planted a seed. You may never adjust them, but something else might have shifted in their life because your agenda was not to get them to become a patient. Your agenda was to share something of yourself with them, with love.

Donny Epstein, D.C.

Love is associated with a biological, biochemical, and energetic reward for establishing a very energy abundant and coherent field between you and another. It adds significant "survival values" — as described by B.J. Palmer, D.C. — to the individual and the collective field of humanity. In love there is so much available energy that there is no longer the need for an individual experience or concept of a "me." There is the pure awareness of the interactions with the loved one as divine gifts, and the unconditional acceptance of the individual as they are.

We can only influence that which we value. We value that which adds more available coherent energy to the system. Interactions that we devalue, dislike, or reject are ones in which energy is lost and the system drops its ability to self-organize in its natural and effective way.

Love is the highest order of adding value to the human experience. A person can only influence that which is valued and respected, including one's pain and disease. Love transcends all of this and must be more than a concept and personally experienced in every interaction.

What would love do? What would love say? How would love talk to practice members, assess them, palpate them, adjust them, consult with them, schedule their visits, listen to them, and be present with them? The answers to these questions are the keys to a thriving practice and life.

The 8 Laws of Chiropractic Success

Brian Kelly, D.C.

As humans we are all expressions of Love. The problem is that we are not always lovable ourselves. We may show up to work and complain, wine, and gossip, forgetting that we are there to love and serve others.

A great way to serve our fellow man is to love them. Certainly, this may be more difficult if the patient doesn't pay their bill and complains the entire time they are in the office. Remember that you are not there to like your patients as much as you are there to serve them at the highest possible level and without being judgmental.

Thom Gelardi, D.C.

Love is all-important. However, true agape love is much different from the pretext of love. Agape love doesn't involve words, it relates to genuine feelings and actions. It means giving the best necessary chiropractic examinations and care you can, regardless of concurrent health problems, or social or financial condition. It means having your cell phone number available and being willing to go out at any time for legitimate reasons. It means referring the practice member to another chiropractor for a second opinion or care if you believe it's in the person's best interest.

Larry Markson, D.C.

Love is the omnipotent force of the universe. It's the energy field I spend a good deal of my time talking about. B.J. [Palmer] once told a class to imagine throwing patients down a flight of stairs (gently) while you're standing at the top of the staircase. As they tumble down the steps, they're getting concussions and their spines are moving all over the place. If you love with intensity as they make their way down, 80% of them will get better.

That's a little farfetched, but that's what love can do. Love heals. Anything you hate, hates you. Anything you love, loves you.

If you really love your patients, if you love your staff, and if you love chiropractic, it's apparent.

Just because being a chiropractor is an easy way to be called *doctor*, or because you can make a decent living without having to drive a truck, doesn't mean you love it. But if you don't love it, your practice will reflect that. When chiropractors don't do well, it's usually because they don't love chiropractic.

Patrick Gentempo, D.C.

In chiropractic terms, I would equate love with passion. If there's no passion, then there's no practice. Chiropractic isn't an easy way to make a living so if you don't love it, it's similar to being in a loveless marriage (see how *that* works!). Love is a key ingredient in order for something to be fulfilling.

Reggie Gold, D.C.

The love angle is part of the "airy fairy" talk by the so-called spiritual people in chiropractic. They're out there talking of love, love, and love. We have Beatles songs for that. Obviously, if you love what you're doing, you'll do a good job. If you love people and really are moved to serve them, you're going to do a much better job than if you're trying to just mechanically approach the spine. When you're adjusting kids, you really care that their subluxations are gone. That part of love obviously is very important.

But I'm not sure these lovey-dovey chiropractors mean that. I think they mean that the laying on of their hands actually brings about a cure. They think, "I love these people and therefore they will get well." They're not talking about chiropractic at all. They're talking about medicine. Spiritual medicine is very effective. Loving what you're doing along with loving what chiropractic truly is makes you more effective.

The beauty of chiropractic philosophy is that you come to understand that *you* do not remove the subluxation. It is so

The 8 Laws of Chiropractic Success

important to understand the fine points of philosophy. If chiropractors aren't trained in those fine points, if they don't really study the philosophy, then they'll think their hands are doing the work.

Kevin Jackson and Selina Sigafoose-Jackson, D.C.'s

Love is certainly the essence of a great chiropractor. Looking back on all the really great and successful chiropractors that we've known, they've all been very loving individuals in their own way. We're not talking about sloppy and sappy people fawning over each and every patient. We're referring to a chiropractor who's in love with the principle of chiropractic, who's in love with diligently teaching the principle of chiropractic, who's in love with performing life connecting adjustments, and who loves people.

Show me someone in love with all the things mentioned above and I'll guarantee they'll be a happy and successful chiropractor. If you're in love with yourself, Facebook, signing people up for money, vacations, and acquiring the things in life ... I'll show you a person who's working harder. What we mean by this is that love transfers immediately from the chiropractor to the patient. If a chiropractor is expressing pure love it becomes like the law of gravity ... it works on everyone whether you believe it or not and it works every time.

Armand Rossi, D.C.

Love is an essential factor in our lives because we love our patients, we love our family, we love God, and it all comes around in full cycle when we're removing interference. Love gets to manifest through people.

Dr. Sid Williams always said, "Give for the sake of giving, love for the sake of loving, and serve for the sake of serving."

It wasn't until recently that I realized this applies to ourselves as well as for others. Loving yourself is a big thing and if you don't love yourself, how can you possibly think other people would want to get care from you?

CJ Mertz, D.C.

Love isn't just a *factor* in chiropractic. Love and chiropractic are *one and the same thing*. I think God is love and God created us through and for love, and led us to create chiropractic to heal our brothers, sisters, and neighbors.

The two golden commandments are: love your God with all your strength, all your heart, and all your soul, and love your neighbor as yourself. For a chiropractor, there isn't a more loving gesture in the world than to provide a solution for someone who is sick and suffering. That, to me, is one of the most Godly acts we can possibly perform.

∞

Terry A. Rondberg, D.C.

Love and service go hand in hand. If we can get out of ourselves and allow Innate to truly flow through us as we serve, we have the pure experience of love. That's the glue and the essence that holds the world together. Love is the essential ingredient and it's everything that God represents.

If we can get out of ourselves and allow Innate to truly flow through us as we serve, we have the pure experience of love.

Unconditional love and unconditional acceptance is an expression of God's love and we have to love ourselves in order to love other people. An intention of mine was to always love and serve my people with the highest integrity and the most intense love I could give them. I hugged, told jokes, gave compliments, encouraged, and tried to inspire all my patients. It all came down to love because if they felt love from me, the practice always flourished.

I think that's true in every walk of life. If you're devoted to service and your intention is to love those you serve, you're fulfilling much of what we were put here to do on this planet.

The 8 Laws of Chiropractic Success

Joe Strauss, D.C.

I don't think love has to be a gushy and "hug all of your practice members" type of thing. That's more emotional and not my type of thing. I think love is a mental attitude rather than an emotion and that mental attitude is something that has to be consistent all of the time. It should come across in your desire to share chiropractic with others and your desire to make chiropractic available. I think that's where I express my love to the community.

Lou Corleto, D.C.

I don't think you can practice chiropractic without the presence of love. You can thrust from your head but you can only adjust from your heart. In your heart is the vibration of love. Empowering the people with an act of vitalism is an act of love. Being willing to face possible rejection in order to help somebody find out about this wonderful thing called chiropractic is an act of love. Having enough compassion for yourself and humanity to keep doing it is an act of love.

Love is vital and is certainly what all living beings need. It's the source of vibration and well-being in our universe. The more you have the courage to give and receive love, the more grounded and powerfully successful your chiropractic practice will be.

Tedd Koren, D.C.

You must first learn to love yourself before you can love others and you must heal yourself before you can heal others.

I don't want to be involved in a practice where everyone is blurting out how much they love one another, high fiving, and giving phony hugs. You have to search the depths of who you truly are and give true love — not make it a game. It has to be a real deep and sincere feeling.

One of the most terrible things I think that B.J. Palmer, D.C. ever wrote was, "I love you because you love the things I love." I never liked or agreed with that quote. The underlying message is, "I love you as long as you keep loving what I love. When you stop loving what I love then you can go to hell."

B.J. did great things and was a great man, but we have to look at him (warts and all) and not copy every little thing he said and did. He made bad mistakes and was an emotional cripple in many ways but on another level, he was a warm, loving, great person and soul.

We don't need to hate him for the wrong things he did and we surely don't need to discard his philosophy because of his mistakes. Nor should we love unquestioningly everything he said and did, or hate people who don't appreciate him the way we do. We have to view things in a balanced way and be open, honest, and admit the painful fact that we may see flaws in B.J. that we also see in ourselves.

Christopher Kent, D.C.

One of the problems with the English language is that we only have one word for love. Many other languages differentiate a spiritual love of all things from a romantic love of an individual and from sexual lust to unconditional acceptance. In other words, we have so many different things that all share the same label that when you say "love" it's kind of hard to hone in on it.

It's a form of love when your intent, focus, vision, and head space are all on seeing the perfection of an individual's manifestation.

Chapter 7

*"What lies behind us and what lies ahead of us are
tiny matters compared to what lives within us."*
– Henry David Thoreau

Law Seven — Giving

David K. Scheiner, D.C.

To give, you must have a sense of abundance within
yourselves. To have a sense of abundance within yourselves
you have to first practice the sacred art of for-give-ness. Forgive
yourself for whatever you did or did not do that you have regret
about. Let it go — it's in the past. Your parents, or whoever, did
what they did and didn't do what they didn't do. People are who
they are. I'm not discounting how you feel regarding traumas that
occurred in your past — those you have to work through if you
so choose. Start with for-give-ness and give up the desire to
resent or punish people. Discover what it's like to be unleashed
in your giving. Make a difference by giving wildly and freely.

When you are overflowing with a sense of abundance from
within and give from that space, it initiates a glow in you; a spark
of life and of light where the universe supplies you with infinite
energy, which you deliver into your practice members.

Notice your relationship with abundance. What's your
motivation with giving and where do you find your sense of
balance with giving and receiving? Feel the joy, peace, and exhil-
aration as you give your gifts of peace, healing, serenity, joy,
happiness, wholeness, and love to those you serve.

First, start by giving yourself the gift of allowing change and transformation to occur within your own self and life. Drop the need to be perfect and develop a self-trust. Allow the possibility of something new and grand to emerge. From this place, you're now free to give for the sake of giving, without looking for anything in return.

D.D. Humber, D.C.

Dr. Sid's Lasting Purpose Principle, as mentioned above, has as a major component, the words "To Give." This is an integral part of one's success as a D.C. student or as a practicing D.C. One must understand and adopt the attitude of being a giving person. Being generous to a fault, giving to others, and to your patients will not only be noticed and appreciated, but will open doors of service like you never dreamed possible.

As a Christian, when I think of giving, I first think of Jesus, my Savior, giving His life on a cross that I might have eternal life. What a blessed promise to those who embrace it. Another example of giving that most people know about and respect whether Christian or not, is that of Mother Teresa, who gave her life in service to thousands and thousands of less fortunate suffering people in the world.

So Chiropractic student and Chiropractor, if you want to succeed...learn to be a giver!

Chuck Ribley, D.C.

It is imperative to have a heart hand and a business hand. With my heart hand I give only to give and without expectations of anything in return. I am also open to receive. The giving and the receiving is like the safety pin cycle. If there is a disruption on either side — the giving or receiving — the relationship is in disharmony, imbalance, and disorder.

The 8 Laws of Chiropractic Success

Janice Hughes, D.C.

Giving is generosity of spirit.
Give of your time, energy,
  and money.
Give to people.
Give attention to others.

Give from a place of abundance and understanding that the more you give and share, the more your own energetic bank account will build.

Tim Young, D.C.

Giving is one of my favorite things to do. I love to perform random acts of kindness. One thing that I have learned on a continual basis is — it is a universal law that it is impossible to give without receiving.

The chiropractic profession, as a whole, has always seemed to adopt a poverty mentality. I talk with doctors all the time who want to feel guilty or make others feel guilty for being successful. My easy answer to this, if you feel guilty for making lots of money, you are not giving enough away.

It is impossible to give without receiving.

Success is all about perspective. I know chiropractors who collect $300,000 per year and feel like they are on top of the world. I also know chiropractors who collect over a million dollars and by being around them or speaking with them you would think the world is against them.

The most successful chiropractors I know are successful not because of how much they have but because of how much they give. Giving of your time is just as powerful as giving money. To the students and young doctors reading this, if you have $5.00 give away $2.50. You will be amazed at how fast your life expands. If you have been in practice for some time, you know what I'm talking about.

The 8 Laws of Chiropractic Success

Neil Cohen, D.C.

The adjustment is a gift that is given and received simultaneously. The chiropractor and patient are in receipt of this precious and unequivocal gift only when a specific and loving adjustment is delivered at just the right moment in time. With this knowledge comes a tremendous responsibility.

We have a wonderful major premise in chiropractic, "A Universal Intelligence is in all matter and continually gives to it all its properties and actions, thus maintaining it in existence." This is your legitimate example to give of yourself because God loves a cheerful giver. Remember that the door you receive through is proportionate to the door you are giving through and that you can never out-give the Giver!

Another golden nugget from the treasure chest of Dr. Sid E. Williams is to give for the sake of giving. You may recognize this as part of the triune of the Lasting Purpose mindset which is, "To Give, To Love, and To Serve," out of your own abundance and without expectation of anything in return. This is intended as sacrificial giving which makes dejection and rejection impossible and has been a brilliant vehicle in structuring my mind.

My challenge to you as a chiropractor, a student, and anyone else who is invested in reshaping humankind is to adopt this mindset as part of a chiropractic paradigm as you make your way through the ever-winding roads of life.

Jessica Harden, D.C.

John D. Rockefeller once said, "God gave me my money...I believe the power to make money is a gift from God...to be developed and used to the best of our ability for the good of mankind." Rockefeller believed that his was entrusted with the responsibility to help people and he was dedicated to ensuring his success went to great causes. Giving does not have to always be in the form of money; it can be in the form of time.

Examine for a moment why some of the most successful

chiropractors in our profession appear to have so much joy and passion for what they do. Is it because they have made great amounts of money? If that were the case, every financially successful chiropractor would be this way, and if you look closely you will find not all are joyfully generous. These passionate entrepreneurs are such because they find pure joy in giving back their time, money, and energy.

If on the road of success you feel depleted of peace and joy, perhaps you are focusing too much on scarcity and forgetting that you as a person are enough and have more than enough to serve. Freely give and relish in the renewed sense of energy and freedom that comes from it.

Paul Reed, D.C.

There is no greater feeling in the world than seeing someone's life light up from something you have given them. The joy, the smile, and the gratitude that is expressed is palpable. Every day in your chiropractic office you get to give the gift of health and full life expression. There is nothing greater or more fulfilling than seeing a patient bounce in the office with a huge smile and joy in their spirit, having just received the care you provided. Principled chiropractic is reconnecting the body and spirit to work in unison.

Principled chiropractic is reconnecting the body and spirit to work in unison.

You must make sure to find other ways to contribute and give to your community. You can do annual food and clothing drives for those in need, patient appreciation days, team sponsors, lectures to groups on different health topics, and so much more. When you find ways to pour into your community with an open heart and expect nothing in return, from my experience, you will be blessed beyond belief.

Brad Glowaki, D.C.

As a chiropractor, you are in the profession of giving. One of the first things you need to learn to give to your patients is value.

"There's no traffic on the extra mile." Give them the opportunity to see the value of chiropractic, beyond its ability to take them away from pain. Give and show them the value of the chiropractic lifestyle and present it with confidence. Your confidence will equate to competence in the mind of your patients. This will lead to greater success for you — the chiropractor — down the road.

Beyond that, constantly look for ways to give more to your patients. "There's no traffic on the extra mile." Always give great service and extra touch points. In my office, for example, it can be as simple as always making personal phone calls to our patients after the first adjustment, showing them that we are an office full of love, caring, and that our intentions are high.

Steve Judson, D.C.

Our gift is our principle, a Universal law, that there is an intelligence in every single person that is perfect although not currently being expressed to its fullest potential. How's your Atlas? That's the single-most important question you must understand as you try to create an awesome life for yourself and the people you take care of.

Atlas subluxations rob life from the body and destroy LIFE expression! The chiropractors gift to humanity is keeping the Atlas clear. This is where the real power resides and the promise of human potential is unlocked. It is not a gift to be nicely wrapped-up and saved for some future holiday season. This is the gift that every man, woman, and child needs and deserves to experience for a lifetime.

Gilles LaMarche, D.C.

St. Francis of Assisi said, "For it is in giving that we receive," Mark Twain said, "To get the full value of joy you must have someone to divide it with," and Bryant McGill said, "Giving is the master key to success, in all applications of human life."

The more you give the more you receive and the less you give the less you receive. How big or how small is the hole you give through? Make it big and also give what you can when you can, whether in time, talent, or treasure.

Like you, I used to resist giving and it was a tiny amount if I gave at all. It took me a long time to realize that by not giving, or not giving freely, I was sending messages to my mind such as "There isn't enough," "I won't get any more," "I might need this for an emergency," "I feel safer with this in my pocket," and so it goes. These, as you know, are all fear-based thoughts and self-fulfilling prophecies.

Guess what? The more you hold on tight, to that old limited thinking, the harder it really is to attract good grades, patients, relationships, success, money, and have it stay in your life. Your scarcity mindset simply won't let it in. So give from a sense of abundance based on what you might have and from your ability to give. If you have $10.00, be willing to give $1.00. If you have little time, be willing to volunteer one-hour per week or per month. Give from your own abundance, whatever that might be, but do start giving.

Ross McDonald and Rebecca Vickery, D.C.'s

Every act of giving changes the world for good. Helping others helps us to find purpose and contentment in our lives when we take an action which benefits another person. Winston Churchill stated, "We make a living by what we get; we make a life by what we give."

Not all giving has to cost financially.

By giving generously in a random act of kindness, you create

The 8 Laws of Chiropractic Success

impactful change for someone else, creating a stronger and more successful relationship with that person. This heightens value and self-worth in both the giver and receiver, which impacts the healing process. That is true success.

Kevin Jackson and Selina Sigafoose-Jackson, D.C.'s

Giving is an essential part of being super successful. Most people, and especially young chiropractors out of school, are simply trying to survive. Naturally, they may lean towards the "getting" side of things. From getting new patients, getting people to sign up, getting bills paid, and all the other forms of getting. People can smell your intentions about getting a mile away.

Have you ever watched a chiropractor at a spinal screening when they're trying to get people to have their spine checked. People in the vicinity of the spinal screening walk as far away from the area as possible or pretend they don't notice the person doing the screening. If the chiropractor simply showed up to the screening or dinner talk simply to "give" as much information out as possible, it literally turns the tables.

We never "ask" for referrals but we have a 100% referral practice. That's simply accomplished by giving. You can never out-give the giver!

Liam Schubel, D.C.

It has been my life experience that the more you give to anything the more you will receive. Any area in your life in which you want more, I suggest you first look at ways to give more. If you are a student and want better grades, give more of your time to studying. If you want to be a master of technique, give more time engaging with it. If you want a more profitable practice, give more of your time to developing solid business systems and creating stronger relationships within your community.

Sales and marketing are vital to any chiropractic business

and the giving mindset is just as important. Have you ever been around a salesperson or marketer that you felt was out to "take" something from you. Whether it was information or money, I'll bet your experience didn't feel good, you didn't want to be in that person's presence, and you wouldn't recommend others to that person's services.

People can generally detect when a person is "on the take." The most successful chiropractic offices look to give people opportunities for a better life through chiropractic. They look to give them education, give them the unique service of LACVS (Location, Analysis and Correction of Vertebral Subluxation), and give them an opportunity to express their lives optimally through an unobstructed nerve system.

People want to buy from and refer to chiropractors whose goal is to give for the sake of giving. There are enough takers in this world today. Start giving and watch the universe respond to you exponentially.

Frederick A. Schofield, D.C.

Giving is not that which you think it is. To give is to receive.

Giving has 3 aspects:

1) Ask and it shall be given unto you
2) Seek and ye shall find
3) Knock and it shall be opened unto you, for you, and onto prosperity

For those that ask, receive and those that seek, find. And those that knock shall receive prosperity. Give the adjustment without the expectation, with love in your heart, peace in your mind, and service with your hands. Give thanks for the blessing that the patient chose your office.

The aspects of Giving:

Give up Something
Give into Something

The 8 Laws of Chiropractic Success

Give Thanks

Give more than you Receive

Give Love

Give Peace

Give Service

Guaranteed you will receive more than you give.

Be Still and Sow and SO IT IS!!!

Daniel & Richelle Knowles, D.C.'s

Give more, serve more, and you'll receive more. In chiropractic and in life, people focus their attention on what they're going to get. I am going to make this much money. I am going to get fifteen new people at this class. I am going to sign up thirty new people at this fair. I need to get more new patients. I need this and I need that ... The focus here is on what I need and want versus what am I going to give. Tony Robbins put it perfectly when saying, "The secret to living is giving."

"The secret to living is giving."

The energy state when you approach a person, event, or situation with what you want to get is completely different than the energy state you're in when giving. If you're out to get something, you'll never be able to give as much. Start each relationship with the focus on how you can help and what you have to give them. Ask yourself the question, "How can I add more value to the other person in the relationship so they have a sense of increase in their life?"

It is a universal law that the more you give and serve, the more you will inevitably receive. The boomerang always returns. Maybe not at the speed you want it too but know it always returns.

St. Francis of Assisi summed it up wonderfully, "Oh divine master, grant that I may not so much seek to be consoled as to console, to be understood as to understand, to be loved as to love. For it is in giving that we receive, it is in pardoning that we are pardoned, and it is dying that we are born to eternal life." Make sure that you give all that you have without looking for anything in return. You will ultimately receive what you deserve for what you've so graciously given.

Brian Kelly, D.C.

How can you give fully and selflessly at the highest level? This is perhaps one of the deepest questions a chiropractor or future chiropractor can ask themselves.

Many chiropractors give fully to their patients at a very high level. However, chiropractic is still a relatively young and small profession, not having completely made it on the proverbial map. For our profession to continue to grow and flourish it is our individual responsibility to also give within the profession.

Professional responsibilities include membership of your State or National Association, contributing to Research (financially or writing research), paying it forward to chiropractic students, or giving your time, talent, or money to chiropractic colleges, and gifting part of your Estate back to the profession. There are many great causes within chiropractic that you can give to and serve with your time or financial contribution.

What would you like your legacy to be in chiropractic? What will your colleagues and family say at your funeral? How do you want to be remembered? We are where we are today in chiropractic because of those who have given before us.

Jason Deitch, D.C.

Giving is one of those interesting concepts that's a paradox. On a basic level, most of you think of giving as transferring something you have to someone else. On the surface, it appears to be a loss when you give to someone.

However, when looking at the concept of "giving" in the context of universal law, you'll see giving has somewhat of a

The 8 Laws of Chiropractic Success

boomerang effect. In other words, in a very non-linear dynamic way, giving of your time, attention, and material things to others, creates a universal energy that returns even more of what you're giving, back to you. It's just one of those things that you have to intellectually understand and trust in order to take the leap of faith that when you give you are creating an opportunity to receive.

Trust that the more you give, the more you'll receive in time. They key is trusting the principle and being patient with the process. You may not receive exactly what you want from the person you give to and in the timeframe you hope to receive it. Trusting the principle, even when it doesn't appear to be working, is the work. Like breathing, giving and receiving are part of universal law.

∞

Amanda & Jeremy Hess, D.C.'s

It's human instinct for us to default to thinking about how life should be fair and that we get what we think we deserve. Think of children and how they automatically say, "Why did he or she get that and I didn't" or "That's not fair, I didn't get anything." We all, from time to time, get caught up in what we're getting in life versus what it is that we ought to be giving.

Zig Ziglar, one of our favorite motivational speakers said, "You can have everything in life you want, if you'll just help enough other people get what they want." The secret of getting what you want is giving and serving the needs and desires of others!

Giving people more than they expect and under promising and over delivering is one of the cornerstones of a successful business, chiropractic practice, and life. Give more than expected. Exceed your practice member's expectations on a regular basis and go the extra mile with your care and your facility. Delivering overall excellence in their practice experience is the kind of giving people have a hard time putting into words. They will however, silently reward you with commitment to care and referrals.

You'll find no greater satisfaction in life than the giving away of your unique talents and treasures.

The 8 Laws of Chiropractic Success

Gerard Clum, D.C.

I was taught about the value of giving for the sake of giving, not giving to get, not giving because somebody will think good of you, not giving because you want others to say nice things about you or remember you with affection, or anything of that nature. You give because you wish to give — period. Yet, I've seen people give money to family members and then get mad because of the way the money was spent. If it's a gift, it's given and it's gone. You let go of it.

Chiropractors are extreme givers in certain ways. The physical interaction you have with a patient during an adjustment is a very giving procedure. But, if you give of yourself and afterwards think the patient didn't pay enough, that's barter, not giving. I do this and you do that and if we're friendly about it we interpret the interchange as giving. That's not what giving is. Giving is free, unfettered, and unencumbered. It's gone as soon as it's given.

Claudia Anrig, D.C.

You can't over-give. Just when you think there's nothing left in you, you just keep on giving. You all have been given a gift, a talent, a blessing, something that is unique to your heart and gives you that special spark. When you can turn around and give of yourself through that gift, you have the potential to touch hundreds of thousands of lives. You certainly can't get burned out from giving.

Patrick Gentempo, D.C.

You have to give every day. If I'm a professional football player in the Super Bowl, what role does giving play in my success during the game? I have to give it all and leave one-hundred percent on the field; I'm going to do everything I can to win. Giving doesn't mean that I don't get paid to play the game. It's a matter of giving the best I have to give and the world will reward me proportional to how good I am.

Larry Markson, D.C.

In all of life, giving is generosity, service, and love — and the more you give, the more you get. Giving plays the exact same role in chiropractic. This is a generous and abundant universe. The more you give to people of your energy and positive intent, the more you will receive back.

Giving is generosity and generosity and forgiveness are the two biggest gifts you can ever give anyone. Giving of yourself to a principle that's higher than yourself can change the chiropractic profession.

Thom Gelardi, D.C.

Giving should be a part of our self-discipline. Some give to causes because they feel pressured by their peers to give. But you need to give wisely and thoughtfully. A major part of a chiropractor's giving should be to chiropractic colleges. No quality college can exist on tuition alone. Chiropractic colleges get little or no government support and little if any foundation support. They're highly dependent on practitioner support.

I believe we should encourage our practice members to support chiropractic causes in ways that don't interfere with the doctor-practice member relationship. Chiropractic is a calling and caring for practice members is a passion.

Sharon Gorman, D.C.

I have given thousands of hours to the chiropractic colleges and state and national organizations. Many times people have asked me, "Sharon, how do you do it?" The more important question is, "Why do I do it?" I do it because at some level I am selfish. I know about the law which dictates the more I give, the more I get in return.

I'm always looking for more and at better ways to give and make a huge difference. I feel good about myself when I am making a difference. I too have come across challenges and I learn more about myself during these trying times by giving than by hanging around worrying about my own needs being met.

You can never out-give the spirit. It's a law. I don't have to worry about it. I keep giving out of my abundance and I keep getting richer. As a child I was told only to give if I knew I was going to get back. I was taught to be cheap and not to trust so I wouldn't be taken advantage of. In my adult life the complete opposite is true. The action of giving in of itself is very rewarding and quite fulfilling.

Christopher Kent, D.C.

Giving tends to imply a one-way stream, when in reality the interaction between a chiropractor and patient or practice member is really an exchange. Whether there's an exchange of money or not, there certainly is an exchange of energy. Indeed, one of the most intimate interactions possible is that of a chiropractic adjustment.

You don't want to be in a headspace where you're thinking, "Well, gee, if I only see two more people today, I'll be able to make my car payment." Some people would say that's greedy, that you should be in a giving mode. I'm saying it's not a matter of giving and taking so much as it is a dynamic exchange to achieve balance. That's the goal. You want to balance, you want to be balanced, and so does the patient.

Joe Strauss, D.C.

I don't "give" chiropractic adjustments to people, because I expect them to reimburse me for that service. I get reimbursement for the adjustments, which makes it an exchange rather than giving. I can exchange an adjustment for some money but my giving is in the area of educating people and sharing with them something that can have a profound effect upon their lives.

The giving in chiropractic involves explaining chiropractic

The 8 Laws of Chiropractic Success

to others, educating them, and giving them information about The Big Idea without any thought of reward.

One of my roles in life is to get as many people to understand chiropractic as I possibly can. I give out information. I give out an idea. I give out a way of looking at life and health. I also give out a way of looking at the function of the body, a way of expressing more of life. That's my giving.

CJ Mertz, D.C.

When we think of the cycle of prosperity, we have to think of giving and receiving. If you give, you shall receive and it goes in that order. Giving is an incredibly important part of one's prosperity because as you give, you open up huge doors of prosperity. Acts of giving are critical because it allows a chiropractor to position himself or herself to receive incredible prosperity.

I've found that with many chiropractors there's confusion between gifting and rewarding. For instance, they'll give something to each person who refers a friend to their office. To me, that's a reward but not a gift. There's nothing wrong with that, but it's not a gift because the person had to do something for you before you did something for them. That means you received something and now you're giving in return.

When we get to the point where we give *before* we receive, it's phenomenal how many doors open for us. As an example, you might give a beautiful and thoughtful gift (not necessarily an expensive one) to patients who come in for six adjustments in a row because you know each adjustment adds to the next.

You also know that the body only heals and corrects by rhythm and so you present a gift to acknowledge those patients who have been coming in for care exactly as they were supposed to.

You give the gift not because of what the patients did for you, but because they did something right and you're praising them for it. When you're truly giving, you'll find that the receiving end of the equation — and I'm talking about your income — literally goes up astronomically. It's a cycle of prosperity.

The 8 Laws of Chiropractic Success

Cathy Wendland-Colby, D.C.

Believe it or not, giving is easier than receiving. Receiving is awkward, uncomfortable, and can feel just downright icky at times. Don't believe me? Ever had someone give you a compliment and you squirmed to offer one back? Queen Elsa tells Princess Anna, "You look beautiful," to which Anna replies, "Well you look beautifuller." Awkward.

The law of reciprocity teaches us that when you give, you shall also receive. And givers absolutely gain. However, some people give with the intention of receiving rather than with the mindset of giving of themselves. That feels like there are ulterior motives, which feels messy and causes people to grow suspicious of the giver who is silently and secretly waiting with their hand out.

> **Help others around you receive, by becoming a gracious giver.**

Help others around you receive, by becoming a gracious giver. Start small; give a smile to a stranger, give unsolicited compliments to acquaintances, give a hug to someone who may not have had any physical touch that day, and when it comes to your patients, give them hope. You may be the only one who does for quite some time.

Terry A. Rondberg, D.C.

Giving is a very positive state of mind and a very positive intention. To be giving of yourself is the highest giving there is. Giving money and other tangible items is charitable and a good thing to do, but being of service and giving of yourself all of the time, surrendering your ego to something greater than you, is truly honorable. Being available and focused, having integrity, and trying to help another human being by giving adjustments are the greatest services you have to offer the world.

The 8 Laws of Chiropractic Success

Armand Rossi, D.C.

The best advice is to do what Dr. Sid Williams always said, "Give for the sake of giving out of your own abundance." You may not think of yourself as being abundant yet, but if you give out of the abundance you do have, it'll hook you back into the gifts of the universe.

One of the most powerful things people can do when they're stuck is to give a gift to someone and never tell anyone they gave it. That's true giving.

Lou Corleto, D.C.

I used to buy into the notion that it's better to give than to receive. At this point of my evolution, I think that's nonsense. The universe requires balance, so receiving and giving in the same spectrum is paramount. The more you're able to receive, the more you're able to give. It's important to keep those channels open and balanced on both ends.

Many people — myself included — have spent a good portion of their lives trying to out-give the giver, so to speak. By doing that, you close the nozzle on the receiving end and end up giving from self rather than from source through self. When you do that, you inevitably deplete yourself mentally, physically, emotionally, and spiritually. When you're open to receiving while giving, you're an open conduit and your supply will keep replenishing.

Tedd Koren, D.C.

You can't truly give unless you feel that you can. Some people are black holes and they feel empty inside, unloved, and in pain. If you feel that way, you can't give. You can sit through a lot of weekend motivational programs where they shout, "You gotta give and you gotta love." But what if you don't really feel you *can* give or that you have anything to give?

If that's the case, you need to simultaneously learn how to give and how to love. Otherwise, you'll be in constant conflict and turmoil and continue being an empty vessel. You must take a hard look at yourself and figure out what it is you need to do in order to heal your emotional wounds and be able to give. We can no longer live our lives on empty slogans. We have to be sincere, honest, and work within the culture we live in.

Jim Dubel, D.C.

God gave me the ability to adjust people regardless of their gender, age, nationality, or religious belief. I give them a secret to better health, the Chiropractic adjustment.

There is an old saying, 'You can't out give the giver.' I feel it's our duty as Chiropractors to give care to anyone in need regardless of their condition or financial ability to pay.

Reggie Gold, D.C.

I practiced with a box on the wall and that shows how I feel about giving. I gave a million dollars to Sherman College and that also expresses how I feel about giving. I learned that giving in those ways makes me happy.

A box-on-the-wall practice can still work and it's the purest form of chiropractic. It allows you to do your job with total freedom because money isn't a factor. If people put nothing in the box, they still receive the same benefit from getting rid of subluxations.

Jim Parker, D.C. and some other people have said that if you don't charge enough money, people won't get well. That's absolute nonsense. You explain to people that their financial situation is none of your business and you trust them to know what to do.

Look at it this way, there's no *right* price for a chiropractic adjustment. Let's say we're dealing with an architect married to an accountant. Maybe they're earning a quarter of a million dollars a year and have no kids. How much can they afford to pay each time they come in?

I advise people, after their subluxations are brought under control, to come in for the rest of their lives for regular care once a week to have their spines checked. In the situation above, the husband and wife are both professionals and earn good money. How much should they pay per visit?

In other words, there is no correct fee. This is what got me out of the fee system and into the box-on-the-wall system. Since there is no proper fee, the chiropractor ought to put a box-on-the-wall and allow people to determine their own fee. I have touched a lot of lives with my suggestion that a box-on-the-wall is a wonderful way to go. Some of the wealthiest chiropractors practice that way and some of the best donors to the colleges and other funds are box-on-the-wall chiropractors.

Some worry that people will rip you off practicing that way or that some won't put money in at all because you don't see what goes in. That's true, some people will rip you off, but then some people will rip you off no matter what you do. If we charge insurance companies and then the insurance company refuses to pay for some reason, what do we do? Go after the patients themselves? With a box-on-the-wall you're totally free from all that crap.

Teri and Stu Warner, D.C.'s

As children, our moms taught us the idea that, "It's better to give than to receive." Although our moms may not have been familiar with the concept on an esoteric level, we've now studied the mechanisms of the universe and how this concept operates through a kind of dynamic exchange. Having experienced this concept first hand, it seems to reason that giving and receiving are different aspects of the same flow of energy in the universe.

There is a universal Law of Giving and Receiving. The Law of Giving says, "The more you give of yourself without expectation of anything in return, the more that will come back to you." Dr. Sid Williams, during our education, reminded us often to "Give for the sake of giving." It became part of our daily mantra. This guiding principle was so important and fundamental to us that when we were new in practice, we would tithe to the church, give back to Life College and other chiropractic causes, and support mission work, before we paid our rent or the electric company. We knew that if we gave enough 'from our abundance,' without any expectation or desire for a return, there would always be a natural energetic exchange where we'd receive back — and we always did! Decades later, this still remains a guiding force in our lives.

On several occasions, we have had the privilege of sharing the stage with Dr. Deepak Chopra. He says, "Practicing the Law of Giving is actually very simple; if you want joy, give joy to others; if you want love, learn to give love; if you want attention and appreciation, learn to give attention and appreciation; if you want material affluence, help others to become materially affluent. In fact, the easiest way to get what you want is to help others get what they want."

Wealth is just as much about what you give as it is what you have. The idea of focusing on being generous as a goal in and of itself, is the key. Don't have the aim be to pat yourself on the back or to strive for admiration from others. Have it be to give just for the mere satisfaction of knowing it made life a little easier for someone else. Tony Robbins once said, "To truly feed your spirit, remember this: The secret to living is giving."

∞

Donny Epstein, D.C.

Giving is natural expression of the previous six laws; Mindset, Vision, Intention, Service, Acceptance (eliminating the experience of rejection) and Love (making rejection irrelevant or impossible).

Service is expressed by the energetics of how these "laws" are experienced and acted upon. The source of the giving must be beyond oneself, as are the sources of Intelligence and Energy. To

The 8 Laws of Chiropractic Success

receive individuals as they are, beyond the hunger to fix them, repair them, judge them, or condemn them, and receiving what they bring to you as a gift, changes the energy dynamics in the field between you and them and your impact upon them.

Ultimately, the gracious receiving of gifts, especially those that are less likely to be experienced as gifts, gives a gift that transforms all.

∞

Billy DeMoss, D.C.

Thou shall give more than is received is the universal rule. When you give love you'll get it back. When you give negativity, you'll get that in return. Being successful in chiropractic means always delivering and giving out of your own abundance and not so you can get something back. Use this principle as a guide and have it deep-rooted in your everyday life.

I was recently at an event where I adjusted hundreds of people for hours and hours. There was no promise of financial reward and most of them didn't even live in the area. I did it because giving a good adjustment and turning them onto chiropractic was more valuable than any monetary reward. Do what you do because you love people and do it because your ability to provide that which so few can becomes the driving force behind it.

John Demartini, D.C.

In my book How to Make One Hell of a Profit and Still Get to Heaven, I debunk the idea of giving because, according to Alfred Marshall, nobody can move a muscle without a motive and that motive is always self-serving.

When we say we're giving, we're actually doing it out of guilt or shame for something in our past or for some hidden agenda in the future. I'd rather throw out the word giving and put in the term fair exchange. When we give service to others, we do it to feel good, because we feel guilty, or because we think it'll give us a marketing boost or something.

The 8 Laws of Chiropractic Success

Chapter 8

"Action is the foundational key to all success." – Pablo Picasso

Law Eight — Action

David K. Scheiner, D.C.

Our final Law is Action. It is the piece of the puzzle that puts the rest of our Laws into motion, igniting the spark of life and infinity itself. When you see the opportunity in your own life to initiate, bring this experience powerfully into being. It is the universe calling you to serve and as Napoleon Hill puts it, "Attack!" You may never get the same chance twice so be bold and relentless in your pursuit of greatness and excellence.

Thoreau once talked about setting lofty goals in the air because that is where they ought to be. He added that we must put foundations under them and I say that those foundations are your empowering action plans. Put your plans into action and do not stop until you've asked every man and woman in your town to be under your care. Then once they are under care let them know about the importance of bringing their children in to be checked for vertebral subluxation merely because they are better off without the interference than with it.

Jim Sigafoose, D.C., created a poster that rubbed many the wrong way although I had it hanging in one of my offices. It read, "Go ahead and leave your children at home so they can experience the same problems you're having for the rest of their lives." Sigafoose,

Sid, Reggie, Pasquale, Santos, Sotille, Parker, Palmer, the contributors in this book, and on and on — all in constant action, motion, and service — rejection-proof, and never idle.

What is your new dream? What do you want your practice to offer the world? Go in the direction of that and break free of the shackles, molds, and constraints either you or another has placed on yourself. Be bold, daring, and deliver your gifts to the masses.

The time to act is now. You do not want to wait until you are on your deathbed and think to yourself, "If I only would have followed my dreams. What would have my life been like then?" Have no regrets in this life. Move to the beat of your own drum. Create movement, momentum, and start now! Say to yourself over and over, "If not me who and if not now when?"

Allow the universe to call you into action in New ways. When that moment that action is available grab it. Share with others what you are out to accomplish and discover. What you already know, you already know. Go and discover the new and the sacred. Hold a mirror up and discover yourself. Don't go to Home Depot and replace the mirror in your bathroom because you don't like what you see in the reflection. It's never the mirror that needs replacing.

This isn't a practice life and it isn't slowing down. Your action is about constant discovery and sharing it with others. You have to feel the urgency and take action — bringing your uniqueness and messages of truth out to the world.

D.D. Humber, D.C.

For years I taught a class at Dynamic Essentials Seminars called *101 Ways to Attract New Patients*. In later years the name of that program was changed to *Action Steps That Empower*. The reason for this change was that almost every idea on attracting new patients required action.

My friends, it is my view that after six decades of Chiropractic involvement in school, seminars, and practice, required action is the ultimate decision maker in your success. You may apply all the previously written laws of success, but without follow through, without action, none will bring about the desired result and you can (no pun intended) take that to the bank!

Chuck Ribley, D.C.

Action for me is the lubrication, the verb of applying esoteric principles into fruition. Thought without action is nil. Action without thought is nil. I am here on this physical plane to take the inspiration from within and express it in a physical way for the betterment of humanity.

Do these principles work! YES! I have created a chiropractic practice of 300-400 patients a day. I have been in politics and served on the Michigan Licensing Board for ten years.

I was one of the co-founders of Life Chiropractic College (now Life University) in 1974 and assisted it to grow into the largest chiropractic college in the world. I assumed the role of board chair at Life University in 2002, leading it through the tumultuous years to once more become the educational leader of the chiropractic profession throughout the world.

There is a quantum field of unlimited possibilities that one can tap into at any time.

Guy Riekeman, D.C.

There are two types of action: action needed for survival and action based on commitment. If you're walking in the woods and a bear comes across your path, you turn into the fastest runner in the world trying to escape. You haven't suddenly become a committed athlete; it's strictly a survival action.

Colin Powell explained the difference very well when he said that commitment is when you're doing the right thing for no other reason than you said you were going to do it, even when no one's looking.

The 8 Laws of Chiropractic Success

You must do the right thing even when nobody's looking. You need to be into committed action. I've seen chiropractors fresh out of school go into their community and put door hangers on every house in the area, or knock on doors and introduce themselves to one-hundred people a day. That's a survival action and as soon as they're out of survival mode, they stop doing it. That's a lot different than the action of committed chiropractors who continue to spread the chiropractic message even when they're long past survival mode.

Frederick A. Schofield, D.C.

Thots and intentions create our Reality, thru space time repetition. Action is the active ingredient that transforms thots and intentions into reality!!!

First you crawl, then you walk, and then you run. Take action on the small things. Small is the next big, get the small idea and the big ideas will take care of themselves.

Action has to do with discipline, self-mastery, and self-awareness. Discipline is not punishment. Discipline is disciplining yourself daily to the truth of your being.

Sensei Shiromo, my Sensei, used to say, "One push-up every day, 365 days a year is better than one time 365 push-ups." Why? because of the discipline it takes to do it daily.

The action is in the small. i.e. Create the four card Monday handouts.

A sower came to Sow (meaning there was an intention. An intention to do something)

1) The first seed fell on the Rocky ground shriveled up and Died

2) The second seed fell on the sandy soil, no roots. When the floods come = destruction

3) The third seed fell forward into the weeds and thorns, the naysayers, the pessimists — leave them behind

4) The last seed fell on the fertile soil and multiplied 30, 60, and 100 fold.

Take Action, go out, and Sow Your Seeds of Health, Happiness, and Prosperity!!!

Be Still and Sow and SO IT IS!!!

Billy DeMoss, D.C.

Upgraded action is hustle and I'm all about the hustle. It's incredibly important to have all the previously mentioned Laws of Chiropractic Success, but hustle is what makes all of these concepts real. Taking massive action to achieve goals is how your purpose in life becomes clear and within your grasp.

Be completely obsessed with turning your goals into action. Get out into the world now and engage others in order to reach your goals. I also want you to realize that inaction in life is failure. No one became successful by remaining stagnant. A still pond always dries up!

Many of you have the certainty in chiropractic but you don't go out and do anything with it. Delivering your message 1:1 and in groups is imperative. We hear the statistics of how many people are under chiropractic care and how many there are still left to reach; it's in the billions! Do your part in educating and taking chiropractic to the masses. The small few cannot carry the entire load alone. Come join us — together we'll take enormous ACTION and move the needle!

Gilles LaMarche, D.C.

Years ago, I learned that action eliminates fear. For you to achieve any level of success, lack of action is never an option; action is an imperative. Many people have ideas, dreams, and passions that they'll never pursue. Some people fear failure and others fear the unknown and I was once one of those people. I became determined for that to change and it changed as soon as

I developed a willingness to take the first step. When I realized I was OK, I then took another.

The truth about 'taking action' is that once you start doing it, magical things begin to happen. Actually, it's not magical at all, it's simply a result of just starting — and anyone is capable of doing that. I'd like for you to please repeat this statement, "If it is to be, it's up to me." For you to succeed as a student or a doctor, multiple actions are required. Inaction cannot be seen as an option.

Brad Glowaki, D.C.

After signing the lease for my first chiropractic office in the small beach town of Seal Beach, CA, I was told I had made a bad decision because I would not be able to pull my new patients out of the ocean. Instead of just sitting around thinking about how that could be true, I took massive action to make that statement false.

Any action beats inaction and action beats thinking.

One of the first steps I took was to do a spinal screening during one of the surf competitions in which my next new patients were *literally* coming out of the ocean.

Any action beats inaction and action beats thinking. Go out and get things done — it's the only way for you to attain your goals. You'll never feel ready but you will always be prepared.

New doctors in practice, you must start spending a minimum of twelve hours a day filled with actions to fill-up your office with people that need your care. Do this and mark my words — you will soon see the fruits of your labor.

Beyond that, when it comes to your patients, understand that the only thing they will judge you by are your actions. While your words are good, your actions will show your intention. Move forward with that in mind always!

The 8 Laws of Chiropractic Success

Amanda & Jeremy Hess, D.C.'s

Some people look at the success of others and often wonder, ask, or question, "How did you get to where you are in such a short amount of time?" The answer is, "It's the cumulative and compounded effect of action." Moving in the right direction over time equals success in any endeavor *every* time.

It is important for you to understand that, in the midst of massive action, there are temporary setbacks of; falling down, getting back up, personal struggle and victory — all happening over a period of time and eventually leading to unbridled success.

Moving in the right direction over time equals success in any endeavor every time.

We clearly remember Anthony Robbins screaming at his seminars, "Take Massive Immediate Action," when referring to dreams, endeavors, hopes, plans or whatever one wanted to accomplish in life. A common theme of the people in the room was fear of failure, fear of uncertainty, and common complacency.

As chiropractors and leaders we need to fight the human habit of just sitting back and thinking about doing things. We often times suffer from a "paralysis of analysis" or fear of moving forward to what we know to be true or what we must do in order to make a difference in our own lives and the lives of others. Many of you get too caught up in the fear of thinking about what people will think of you! How can you get out in the community and build a practice if that's what is driving you?

Chiropractors are inherently different in their choices, education, and what they stand for. In most cases their thinking is diametrically opposed to the way the world thinks and acts. Never let that that hold you back! Take Massive Immediate Action on your Goals, Dreams, and Vision for your life and your chiropractic practice, while understanding humanity needs you now more than ever!

The 8 Laws of Chiropractic Success

Chiropractors in practice for many years are hit with the temptation of complacency. The poison of success has you resting on your laurels and far too many of our fellow seasoned D.C.'s become content after a few years of serving. How often are you doing outreach like you did when your first opened in your community? How excited are you to teach chiropractic to your practice members on their regular visits or during your "Doctor's Report?" How motivated is your team? Know that their willingness to serve rises and falls according to the attitude, gratitude, and motivation of the leader within the chiropractic office.

Action is simply forward motion, in a positive, pre-determined direction that will get you the results you want to obtain! How much "Forward Motion" have you, your team, or your entire office had recently? How are you measuring your motion or action? Who is holding you accountable? Who, in your inner circle, is rooting you on and is there for you when you stumble and fall? All of **The 8 Laws of Chiropractic Success** are interrelated, but without action they are simply words you're reading on a page. Today, we challenge each of you to Take Massive Immediate Action!

Jim Dubel, D.C.

Anyone can sit in their office with the greatest intention to change the world with Chiropractic. Like having the best mouse trap, if no one knows you have it, it does not catch mice very well.

Chiropractic and its philosophy is what sets the profession apart from any other form of healthcare known to man. We are separate and distinct from all other professions. It is our philosophy that enables us to stand out. "Get the Big Idea and all else will follow." It is the biggest thing I know.

Every Chiropractor needs to get out and sell themselves. You need to take action in whatever way you feel works best for your community. Different examples are; health talks, meeting prospective patients at health fairs, and telling the Chiropractic story to anyone who can and will listen. Sitting behind your desk doesn't get it done. Get your butt in gear and get out of your fear of talking to people about Chiropractic.

Cathy Wendland-Colby, D.C.

Goals without action steps are just dreams. Action steps without goals — now that's a nightmare!

You can read and re-read all of the knowledge shared by the many leaders who have contributed to this book. And you will certainly be better for it. What's paramount is the next step, the critical and most often overlooked work that comes next. Lay out your goals, map out the steps you'll need, and then take action.

Take massive action. This is not the time to be modest or hide your capabilities from the world. If you want better, do better. Have the courage to ask for what you want and then go after it like your life depends on it. Because it does.

It is only when you have goals and action steps that you get to create the reality you want.

Your life is your gift from God. What you do with it is your gift back.

∞

Jason Deitch, D.C.

All of the ideas in this book and principles of success that have stood the test of time are all "ideas" until you put them into action. Action is the enzyme or catalyst for success. You can't expect something good to happen if you're not taking action to move in the direction of your dreams.

Action is your way of showing the universe you're serious about what you want. Action is the way you learn, grow, and improve. Action is the way you accelerate your success. A key factor to achieving success is consistently taking the right actions over time. You should remember the mantra from one of the world's top brands for competitive athletes to "just do it." In other words, if you want to win, you must take action. When will you start and what will you do?

The 8 Laws of Chiropractic Success

Paul Reed, D.C.

Behind every successful person you will see not only action, you'll see MASSIVE action. Action is the key ingredient in your ability to get stuff done. I feel that this has been an instrumental element in my ability to accomplish things in my life. Whether it was my college athletic career, marriage, or business, action has given me the edge needed to do more, go further, and punt when needed. It allows me to move through opposition and be laser-focused in order to get stuff done — Period!

Unfortunately, many of you either do not have BIG enough goals, dreams, and desires or you spend your time procrastinating on the details. You're thinking too much and not moving enough; waiting for the perfect stars to align. I'm here to tell you to just GO because done is much better than perfect.

You know you have big enough goals and dreams when you're completely consumed with so much passion and knowledge that you can't sleep. It's pulling at you in your sleep to get to know it more intimately and in order that you create more of it.

Just go ahead and take some action on whatever it might be that you're wanting to get done. Once you're out moving, that sense of accomplishment will pull you with increased energy and excitement knowing that you're close to the triumph! Keep on Keeping on my friends!!!

∞

Tim Young, D.C.

One of my favorite Sigafoose talks is one where he said, "You can stand on the hood of your car holding the keys and scream into the air, I believe this car will start, I believe this car will start, and never actually get in the car and put the keys in the ignition. Your intention, belief, mindset or philosophy on life mean absolutely nothing without action."

Without action nothing happens and there will be no success. This has become quite the problem with some of the new doctors coming out of school. They took action to get their degree and now they expect to be rich because of a title. I have some very important news for all of you. I don't care if you just graduated or have been in practice for twenty years; you have to show up, every day, and take action.

I tell young docs who are trying to start a practice, take one thousand business cards and hand deliver, one at a time, every card. Meet one thousand people. When you get thru that one thousand get a thousand more. You continue to do that until you are seeing one-hundred patients per week. The most important lesson I can teach you about action is that this process ought to never stop. When you stop, so does your success. Success is not something you achieve. Rather, it is something you become.

Daniel & Richelle Knowles, D.C.'s

Henry Ford said, "You can't build a reputation on what you're going to do." Action is fundamental. We can have a vision, we can have a mind-set, we can own our philosophy, and we can deliver our incredible technique. If we sit around and talk about it, pray about it, meditate about it, or visualize it, never getting off the couch to do something, nothing is going to happen. It's in the DOING that has what you think about brought about. People spend much time over analyzing things. The time is right, the circumstances are perfect and the conditions are ripe for you to take action — NOW! Don't allow anything, including yourself, to keep you from moving forward.

It's in the DOING that has what you think about brought about.

Successful people are constantly moving. Sure they make mistakes, but they never quit. Done is better than perfect and improved upon execution keeps you moving forward. The pathway to success involves taking massive, refined, continued, and determined action. They key to it all my friends is positive thinking combined with positive action.

As chiropractors, let's do something now that shifts humanity for the better!

The 8 Laws of Chiropractic Success

Steve Judson, D.C.

Talk is cheap, planning is frivolous, and goals are road blocks unless you devise a strategy and put it into massive action. When you know what you have to give and who you serve, you're able to have a concise laser-focused vision. Similarly, when you know your outcome, you're able to connect to your purpose, the reason WHY you do what you do.

The beauty is that there is no one who has the potential to clear an Atlas the way a chiropractor does! Hone in on and master your craft. Your vision will ultimately be achieved through action. Dr. Sid Williams taught us to plan to work and work our plan. There's literally no other way. Hard persistent work is the only way to grow and achieve anything in life. After all, it is your one and only life. LIVE WITH PASSION and LIVE CLEAR!!!

Kevin Jackson and Selina Sigafoose-Jackson, D.C.'s

You hear a lot these days about taking massive action to get massive results and of course that's true to a certain degree. We think we need more correct action in the chiropractic setting. More chiropractic action. James Sigafoose used to always say, "You do too much." He meant we were trying too hard, saying too much, and wanting it too badly. These are all symptoms of living from the outside in. He went on to explain that we need to let Innate run the show.

When someone gets adjusted, let them know that their body will take over and get the job done. You don't have to rub on it, take a bunch of vitamins, or stretch it. Simply find it, fix it, and let Innate do the work.

Correct action makes a chiropractic office work. Learn correct action more than massive action. Some of the best ways to learn correct action are by reading a great chiropractic book, getting a great chiropractic mentor, or simply getting in touch with yourself through the sacred art of meditation.

∞

Sharon Gorman, D.C.

It all boils down to action. Although mindset, vision, and intention are important, action is where the rubber meets the road. I have learned over the years that it is impossible to put out energy without it coming back.

You've heard those stories about the chiropractor who puts an ad in the local paper and new patients start calling their office. You come to find out that the ad was never published but the phone starts ringing anyway. How does that happen? They meant to put the ad in the paper but were just too busy and forgot. Their intention and mental energy was put out (action) and a Universal Ad was placed. I love to build brand new practices this way.

I use up all the time I am in the office as an opportunity to be in and of action. The action might be seeing patients, training staff, or implementing procedure. The action might be to actively pursue marketing leads, set up lunch and learns, or create an in-house marketing campaign. My focus is always on creating action and that's where I want yours to be too.

Life is motion. I am always keeping in alignment with life and therefore I'm always in motion. I keep myself so busy that I don't have time to worry. In this way, I become busy seeing patients! It's a game I like to play with myself. Many chiropractors, students, and associates need to create constant opportunities to stay busy so they can become more successful. Get in action and create momentum.

By being active, we see ourselves as more successful, we feel more successful, and we create greater success. Your decisions and actions dictate your destiny — every time!

Teri and Stu Warner, D.C.'s

The path to Massive Practice Success is found by honing your mind, body, and spirit. Make sure you're aligning all three by regularly setting and accomplishing goals for each. Take care of

The 8 Laws of Chiropractic Success

yourself by receiving adjustments, making healthy food choices, exercising, practicing yoga, meditating, and getting proper sleep. If both your emotional mind and physical body aren't in shape, you'll be too exhausted to ever act on and achieve your true practice goals. Lots of people set good intentions, have good ideas, and like to talk about things, but the people who are actually successful are the ones who take action and execute.

In practice, we find it's useful to combine large massive action events (hosting a Kids Day America / International event, building relationships with the media for TV, print, or radio campaigns, hosting a Children's Health Expo or Walk / Run for Children's Wellness) with smaller strategic daily actions (giving new patients an office tour, putting a mirror behind the front desk to ensure the staff always answers the phone smiling, greeting all patients by name, and having water and organic snacks in the office). Putting these two types of actions together will always funnel a healthy stream of new patients through your door.

> **Remember to make people feel BIG by empowering them to do more, be more, and have more.**

Whatever you do, always remember to make people feel BIG by empowering them to do more, be more, and have more. We have the responsibility to educate and adjust as many people around the globe as possible. B.J. Palmer, D.C. told us, "You HAVE in YOUR possession a sacred trust. Guard it well." We have a huge job to do and in order to do it we need to take massive action! People don't know what they don't know, so it's up to us to get out into the media and educate them. Don't let the butterflies in your stomach or your other fears stop you. Be led by your passion, commitment, and purpose instead.

A banner that hangs at our gym reads, "It's You vs. Yesterday." The goals you set today are the results you'll achieve tomorrow. Never forget how powerful chiropractic is. With great knowledge and power comes great responsibility. Go take action and make tomorrow count!

The 8 Laws of Chiropractic Success

Neil Cohen, D.C.

Success in practice, academia, and life can only come from planned out action. Our major premise specifically speaks about actions, "A Universal Intelligence is in all matter and continually gives to it all its properties and actions, thus maintaining it in existence."

Principle two of thirty-three talks about the chiropractic meaning of life and the expression of that life in action, ultimately because it is motion that's necessary for life. Where there is no motion or movement there is no life. Dead things won't move on their own because they are lacking intelligence within. These first two Chiropractic Principles magnificently represent massive coordinated action.

The secrets to successful actions are; 1) The determination to attain your goals accompanied by well thought out strategies and 2) The appropriate execution on those goals.

Haphazard action may or may not keep your head above water, whereas deliberate action will effectively lead you to the highest degree of collateral in reaching your desired goals.

Faith in chiropractic business is not enough. Scripture declares that faith without works is dead. Go to work and energize your practice and your Life. Work tirelessly during your academic experience and you'll be led on a life path of fulfillment and attainment you never thought possible even in your wildest dreams.

Go now and devise a strategic outline of your planned action steps and you'll be certain to fully realize the perfect prophetic vision that God has planned for your magnificent Chiropractic Life!

∞

John Demartini, D.C.

If you don't get off your ass you'll get a sore ass. You have to take action because without it nothing happens. It's said that if you want to get something done, give it to a busy person because busy people get more things done.

Parkinson's Law states that any space and time that isn't

filled with high priority things will be consumed by low priority things. People who take action and are inspired by what they do constantly identify what their priorities are and they keep filling their day with highest priority activities.

When I first got into practice, I did a little of everything, including reports, paperwork, and just trivial stuff — all the $15 and $10-an-hour jobs. I quickly realized the most important thing I could do would be to get up in front of a group of 100-200 people and share a message.

I started getting out there generating tons of patients while someone else did the other stuff in the office. If I gave a twenty-minute speech before sixty people at a breakfast club and I got five new patients out of it and each new patient was a $3,000 case, that was a $15,000 speech.

If I'm in the office doing a report and making $400 dollars an hour, I'm diluting myself. I have to always keep delegating lower priority tasks and follow Parkinson's Law and Pareto's Principle to focus on the highest priority activities to produce the most and see the greatest number of people in the world.

Joseph Durant put Pareto's Principle on the mark originally when he said, "Twenty-five percent of what you do gives you seventy-five percent of the results." Some people call it the 80-20 rule and some the 90-10 rule. Whatever the figures, you have to find out what's most meaningful for you and do those things that are most important.

That's why I'm traveling and speaking today. In the last 30 years, I've reached over 6 billion people through radio, TV, various media, movies, and all the different things that I've done.

∞

Claudia Anrig, D.C.

Action is the energy you put toward achieving your goal. With anything in life, you have to initiate some mental or physical energy to create movement. The action component is the chemistry you provide in order to get a reaction. While your goal might be to grow your practice, if you don't put action toward that goal, don't go complaining about the outcome!

Many people have numerous goals and visions, but they never get going, they don't get out of bed ready for action every day of their lives. They can't blame anyone else if they don't manifest their goals and visions because *they* must be the initiators of the action.

Gerard Clum, D.C.

Action animates everything. All of the Laws we've talked about so far — mindset, vision, giving, intention, rejection, service, love, and action — are part of a chain. If any of the links are broken, the kinetic chain doesn't work, the system shuts down, and nothing gets accomplished.

Dr. Sid Williams once said that work will win when wishing won't. That was the principle I was taught as a young guy: until you put something into action, it's all talk, rhetoric, and theory. It may be all right but it's not real until you put action behind it.

Larry Markson, D.C.

Success is a thought first, a vision second, and then lastly an action step that's in harmony and sync with the original thought. Thought plus action creates the feeling and the emotion. The emotion opens the door between the conscious mind and the subconscious mind.

A thought plus action equals a feeling, which creates success and attracts those things you want into your life. So many chiropractors ask me to tell them what to do but it's never a matter of me *telling* them what to do. It's a matter of them thinking a certain way, and then doing the correct thing, which gives them that right feeling. That's what creates the results.

Thom Gelardi, D.C.

Dreams, prayers, and visions are good only when followed by action. When you pray, move your feet. The universe helps those who help themselves. The universe will judge the sincerity of our intentions by the intensity of our effort. If you put in thirty hours a week caring for practice members, you should put in another twenty hours in business-related and practice-building activity.

Janice Hughes, D.C.

This is where the rubber meets the road. You can have the ideas and intentions, yet without some level of action, you aren't putting the wheels of success into motion. The more consistent the action is the more you will keep moving down the road and down the path of success.

What stops most people at this stage of the success path are the ideas or expectations that change requires massive actions coupled with all the emotions and fears that this brings up. People see the chasm or divide from where they are now to where they need to be and are afraid of the large leap or energy it will take to create the necessary change to get there.

An alternate approach does exist. I ask my clients to focus on their next simplest action step. Not the 'big' step that could create massive change. Simply the next easy simple step. This is the Principle of Kaizen. By starting with something simple, allowing your brain to say, "Oh I can do that," you automatically get in motion. You are now in and of action and can continue that one simple step. Before you know it you easily take another step.

Simple actions in Chiropractic build incredible careers and even more amazing lives!

Enjoy this Maxwell Maltz quote with me, "Often the difference between a successful man and a failure is not one's better abilities or ideas, but the courage that one has to bet on his ideas, to take a calculated risk, and to act."

The 8 Laws of Chiropractic Success

Tedd Koren, D.C.

Action is what repairing the world is all about. You can't just wish it; you have to make it real. Just having fluffy feelings won't get it done. You have to put motion behind what you're doing.

A lot of people wish for world peace but if they don't stand up and take action, if they don't do the necessary work, what they're left with is what they started with: a wish.

The same applies to chiropractors who wish for a thriving and successful practice. It's the old adage of hanging out the shingle when you open a new office. Do you just put the shingle out there and wish that people will see it and walk in? Do you open your office and sit by the telephone hoping it will ring (and when it does, the person's calling to collect the overdue electric bill?)

You have to get off your butt and pound the pavement and don't walk back into your office until you've made connections with multitudes of people in your area who now know you and where you're located.

∞

CJ Mertz, D.C.

Action relates directly to success. Compare two chiropractors, one who sees seven hundred patient visits a week and one who sees only seventy. They may be taking very similar actions when it comes to adjusting, examining, reporting, etc. But look closely and you'll see a massive difference in intent, trust, and speed, all of which are related to action.

Action and the very delivery of action allow chiropractors to reach their fullest potential and be able to serve as many people as they desire. Almost all actions come down to skill. Action therefore is a direct expression of your current level of skill and your skills can improve. As your skills improve, your actions increase. When actions are based on intention, speed, and trust, practices grow. It's a law!

∞

Lou Corleto, D.C.

Without action, things don't move. Action is necessary in order to get force in motion to make anything happen. We've all heard the saying, "Build it and they will come." Sure, that's a great concept but if they don't know that you've built it, they can't find it and receive what you have to offer.

On the practical level, action is marketing yourself so people will know you're there to provide them whatever services you offer. Be proud of your uniqueness and don't try to imitate others. There are many other chiropractors in my area, yet we are completely different and unique.

Our actions let people around us know we exist. When they come in to see us, they get to know who we are and the uniqueness we possess. Our actions should be directed towards constantly working on our skills, our understanding of the principles of vitalism, our ability to deliver the wonderful chiropractic message, and empowering other people. Don't just sit around. Take action.

Joe Strauss, D.C.

The action I want to do in my community is to give people chiropractic care. I don't want to be in the local Lion's Club because the time I'd spend there would take away from the time I could be thinking about chiropractic, writing about chiropractic, communicating chiropractic to people, or putting my hands on people's spines. Our actions have to be in the area of chiropractic.

Terry A. Rondberg, D.C.

Being grateful takes action. Being of service takes action. Intention means nothing without action. Whatever we have in our life that we're grateful for or that we want to serve, in order to make it a reality we have to take it to the next step and level, which is action.

Liam Schubel, D.C.

You cannot think yourself into success. While thinking is vitally important, actions are the manifestation of those thots. One of the most common traits of successful chiropractors and students is persistent action. Everybody has things that they would like to achieve in their lives. It is action however that separates those who talk about what they want from those that go out and make their dreams a reality.

Successful people don't always succeed on their first try at something. As a matter of fact, many people fail many times before finding the combination that unlocks their dreams. Some people focus on those failures, become depressed, and quit before ever reaching their potential. Success comes from acknowledging that failure is part of the learning process. You learn from failure, change your approach, and take persistent action again until you achieve your goal.

Persistent action is truly the great equalizer in life. If you are able to recognize obstacles and adversity as the universe questioning you as to how badly you desire something, then you find a way to take persistent action no matter what. In our business system group Schubel Vision Elite, it is wonderful to see chiropractors light up when they learn that business is not something mystical. They are amazed when they find out that there are definite action steps that make what they thot were impossible obstacles, "Easy!" Never let anyone tell you that something is impossible just because they have not found a way to make it happen.

All chiropractic students and chiropractors in the world could be outrageously successful if they only knew *exactly* what they wanted and refused to quit until they achieved their goals. Chiropractic is crucial to the transformation and evolution of the planet because it unlocks human potential. Knowing this, we have the moral obligation to share this message successfully with the world. Every persistent action that we take in line with this moral obligation will bring us closer to the success we all deserve.

The 8 Laws of Chiropractic Success

Ross McDonald and Rebecca Vickery, D.C.'s

Reading this book is the first step to making changes in your life. However, the glue which holds all these principles together is action. Without doing anything with what you are learning, you are procrastinating and procrastination is the enemy of success! Being successful is not a necessity but a choice. Taking action is a necessary decision you must make to be successful.

Action is movement, the energy to transform ideas into application and success. Only through taking action can information actually be made to be useful in your life. Actions facilitate eliminating bad or recurrent habits in your life while the practice of taking action ultimately leads to transformational change and the formation of new habits and values in your life leading to success and significance.

Brian Kelly, D.C.

Visualization of what you want to see actualized in your life is an important first step. Visualize a remarkable life and an incredible chiropractic practice. Taking massive action, they will move at a great speed towards actualization.

If you want to see more new patients, you can visualize them, conceptualize them, and they will most likely show up. If, on the other hand, you went out into your community and did a spinal screening and put your hands on 150-200 people, with a highly trained staff and a refined follow-through procedure, a large number of these people will show up in your office the following week.

If you desire to be a master chiropractic adjuster; decide it, visualize it, and affirm it. Then go work the next forty years to refine and master your technique.

Some of my chiropractic clients have had dramatic changes in their practice and life by getting up, getting out, getting motivated, and acting upon those specific things we identified they needed to. In contrast, procrastination, contemplation, exaggeration, and hallucination will get you nowhere.

As Nike says...Just Do It!

Patrick Gentempo, D.C.

There's an old B.J. Palmer quote that reads, "Life is motion, motion is life, and the lack of motion is death." Action is movement and movement is a part of the universe. Everything moves. When there's a lack of action you have stasis, which is when you're dying. You can't say you're going to stand where you're standing and try to keep things the way they are. Either you're moving toward illness or you're moving towards wellness right now and there is no squatting. You're going one way or the other.

If you're taking action to promote health, you're going to move in a positive direction. If you're not taking action on that, the second law of thermodynamics and a Law of the Universe called entropy will take over and move you towards disassociation, disintegration, disease, and loss of health.

Jessica Harden, D.C.

There are those people that consciously choose to do nothing, not necessarily because of laziness, which has an obvious solution; but the person is paralyzed by either the choice of where to begin or due to the fear of rejection. To break through this paralysis or rejection, you must choose to do something daily!

Perhaps you have been hit with a difficult situation or maybe you need to make some change in the office or home. Make the daily choice to do something. Simply stand up and put one foot in front of the other. As Vince Lombardi said, "It is a game of inches." Don't look at all of those yards ahead of you. Keep your nose down and celebrate the inches you have pushed through. When you do finally lift your head up you'll be surprise by how many yards you've traveled.

The 8 Laws of Chiropractic Success

On the other hand, there are those people who are too busy. Not all busy people are producing and not all are producing successfully. If just doing something all the time guaranteed success, many more would come by success easily. Being *busy* is so easy to do. Being *productive* requires strategy. Actions should be filtered through your vision. Ask yourself the question, "Is what I am doing bringing me closer to my vision for my life or further away?" If further, you either need to stop doing it or delegate it to someone else.

Have you ever felt as though you never had enough time to get things done? If so, keep in mind that it is not a time problem; It is a priority problem. Prioritize the things you need to do and execute on those that serve your vision the greatest.

Never forget that you have the same amount of time as everyone else. It is what you choose to do with that time that makes all the difference. Get up an hour earlier so you can get in a workout. Cut ten minutes off that daily workout so you can follow up on a lead. Delegate to a team member to run deposits to the bank so you can get an extra half-hour of family time. These are all small decisions and add up to an hour and forty minutes of reassigned time towards potentially refueling yourself. It may help you to produce more or you may simply be more available to the things that matter most. Take action and remember to constantly filter those actions through your vision.

Donny Epstein, D.C.

Always take conscious action consistent with the prior 7 laws, and observe, experience, and assess the action as to your effectiveness in meeting your highest objectives.

Action must be guided, conscious, deliberate, coherent, and aligned with the needs of the person you are serving. This can liberate his innate expression to be a more energetically resourced torch holder for his future, the future of those he will directly influence, and ultimately for a more coherent and connected humanity.

"Never doubt that a small group of thoughtful, committed citizens can change the world. Indeed, it is the only thing that ever has." – Margaret Mead

About the Contributors

Claudia Anrig, D.C.

Dr. Claudia Anrig has been in full-time chiropractic practice since 1981. She is the founder of Peter Pan Potential, the first pediatric chiropractic community outreach program. Claudia mentors chiropractors to grow their family wellness practices through her Generations coaching program. She is a former president and board member of the ICPA. Dr. Anrig's Volume One Pediatric Chiropractic textbook was the first of its kind and the fastest selling textbook in chiropractic. www.drclaudiaanrig.com

Arno Burnier, D.C.

Dr. Arno Burnier is a renowned chiropractor and international public speaker on chiropractic, life, health, healing, and wellbeing. He has been married over 35 years to his extraordinary wife Jane and is a father and grandfather. Arno is a mentor, coach, and teacher to countless doctors of chiropractic and students around the world. His impact and influence in the world of chiropractic, health, and healing is significant. www.cafeoflife.com www.mlsseminars.com

Gerard Clum, D.C.

Dr. Gerard (Gerry) Clum, a 1973 graduate of Palmer College. He held academic positions at Palmer and at Life Chiropractic College in Marietta, Georgia before being appointed President of Life Chiropractic College West in 1981 where he served as President and Chief Executive Officer for thirty years before retiring in January 2011. Dr. Clum currently serves as the Presidential Liaison for External Affairs at Life University in Marietta, Georgia. He also serves as the Director of The Octagon, a "think-tank" addressing matters of health, health care, and contemporary perspectives on Vitalism. www.life.edu

Neil Cohen, D.C.

Dr. Neil Cohen is a 1986 graduate of Life Chiropractic College in Marietta, GA. After running a successful practice in south Florida for more than twenty-eight years, Neil began his tenure as Executive Vice President of Sherman College of Chiropractic in March 2014. Deeply invested in the founding principles of Chiropractic, he has been a Board Member of principled organizations such as the Southern Chiropractic Association and the Florida Chiropractic Society. He has spoken on four continents as a platform speaker, motivating and inspiring those within the Chiropractic profession to join him in ridding the world of chronic subluxation, whereby allowing the full expression of Life and Health. www.sherman.edu

Cathy Wendland-Colby, D.C.

Through her YouTube channel, websites, mentoring programs, and stage presentations around the world, Dr. Cathy Wendland-Colby has empowered over five-million women and families to make healthy choices for their pregnancy, birth, parenthood, and for their family's health.

She is a 1999 graduate of Life University, holds licenses in three states, has two practices in Woodstock, Georgia, is adjunct faculty at Life University, and mentors students and new docs every day in her offices. Cathy recently launched the "Women Speakers Club" Private Facebook group, the "Find Your Voice" 30-Day Challenge on BrandingYourCommunication.com and the women's speaker directory which can be found at www.Book MyNextSpeaker.com

Lou Corleto, D.C.

Dr. Lou Corleto is a Vitalistic Chiropractor, Certified High Performance Coach, Retreat Facilitator, Adventurer, Author, and

Global Humanitarian Mission Leader. Lou graduated with honors from Life Chiropractic College in Marietta, GA in 1992 and has adjusted the Monks in Tibet and served children in orphanages in Brazil. Lou is a brilliant innovator and communicator, expressing everything he says and does through his heart. www.loucorleto.com

Jason Deitch, D.C.

Dr. Jason Deitch is a Doctor of Chiropractic, Author, Speaker, and the founder of AmpLIFEiedLiving, a social media content publisher for inspired healthy living used by thousands of health care professionals around the world — reaching an average of 40 million positive impressions per month. He is the co-author of Discover Wellness, How Staying Healthy Can Make You Rich, as well as the founder of the Discover Wellness Center, an emerging leader in cutting edge wellness care. www.discoverwellnesscen ter.com www.amplifeied.com

John Demartini, D.C.

Dr. John F. Demartini is a chiropractor, human behavioral specialist, educator, and international authority on maximizing human awareness and potential. His studies encompass more than 270 different academic disciplines including research into most of the classical writings of both Orient and Occident. To date, he has taught his principles and methodologies in over sixty countries and has students in most countries across the world. Dr. Demartini is founder of the Demartini Institute, originator of the Demartini Method, and he has homes in the United States, Australia, and on The World of ResidenSea. www.drdemartini.com

Billy DeMoss, D.C.

Dr. Billy DeMoss is an energetic and passionate international speaker who has been a chiropractor and leader within his community for over three decades. He is the founder of the Dead Chiropractic Society (DCS) and in 2008 decided to expand DCS by founding California Jam, where he invites world-renowned experts in chiropractic, public health, and global sustainability to educate and empower people from around the world who find natural solutions more attractive than harmful man-made ones. His mission for Cal Jam is simple: awaken, empower, action. www.demosschiropractic.com www.californiajam.org

Jim Dubel, D.C.

Dr. Jim Dubel is a Palmer graduate and opened Health in Hand Chiropractic in New Jersey with his wife, Babs, at his side in 1980. Ten years later they started the New Beginning for a New Future Chiropractic Philosophy Weekend, known best as New Beginnings. From its humble beginnings, the event has grown under their direction and guidance. It is now one of the premier chiropractic philosophy events in the nation, drawing hundreds of chiropractors as attendees and attracting the best of the best in chiropractic philosophy presenters. New Beginnings is celebrating its 25th anniversary this year. www.nbchiro.com

Donny Epstein, D.C.

For more than four decades Dr. Donny Epstein has been impacting millions with models of healing and living, tailored to a person's unique innate signature. In addition to his four books, eleven universities have spearheaded academic research and nearly one-hundred peer reviewed articles have been published consistent with his personalized energetic disciplines.

Donny's methods include the Network applications in chiropractic, Somato Respiratory Integration, EpiExchange — an energetic discipline based on optimizing available energy in the field around the body, EpiPerformance which includes the energetic dynamics between people in organizations, and the Pain Integration Experience. His evolving approach, EpiEnergetics, encompasses his Reorganizational models of healing and living to power seekers for the extraordinary. www.EpiEnerget ics.com, FB @epsteindonny, Instagram @donny.epstein

Thom Gelardi, D.C.

New York native Dr. Thom Gelardi graduated from Palmer School of Chiropractic in 1957. After graduation he moved to Gaffney, South Carolina and developed a very successful practice while raising a family of five children. In 1973 Gelardi founded and became the first President of Sherman College of Chiropractic in nearby Spartanburg. He lead the progress of the school for nearly three decades, serving as President until 1997 and later as a member and chair of the board of Trustees from 1997- 2002. Dr. Gelardi has traveled throughout the world as a lecturer and has written extensively on chiropractic philosophy. www.sherman.edu

Patrick Gentempo, D.C.

Dr. Patrick Gentempo is the family centered, simplistic, and purpose-driven founder and CEO of Action Potential Holdings, Inc. He is well-known and respected in the world of health, wellness, and business. While practicing as a chiropractor, he co-developed innovative diagnostic technologies, received multiple patents, and built a considerable international business which he led as CEO for over twenty years. Academically, Patrick is on the post-graduate faculty of multiple chiropractic institutions and has been published numerous times in peer-reviewed and popular journals. He regularly lectures to business owners, health providers, and entrepreneurs. Dr. Gentempo lives with his wife and three children in Park City, Utah.
www.patrickgentempo.com www.actionpotentialholdings.com

Brad Glowaki, D.C.

Dr. Brad Glowaki is an internationally known and experienced speaker who teaches about new patients, concussions, personal injury, and more! Dr. Glowaki has helped thousands of chiropractors around the world become better communicators, serve more people, and be more successful. Dr. Glowaki is still in practice in Seal Beach, California where he lives with his wife and four kids. www.glowakichiropractic.com www.newpatient maven.com

Reggie Gold, D.C., Ph.C.

Dr. Reggie Gold was the world's leading authority on chiropractic communications. The techniques he developed have proven successful for thousands of chiropractors. Reggie graduated Summa Cum Laude as class valedictorian from Palmer College in 1957, and he served in various capacities in state and national organizations during his career. He founded one Chiropractic College, assisted in the founding of another, taught philosophy at three colleges, and lectured at most of the others. On top of all this, he managed to run one of the most successful practices ever — known at a time and in a place where the practice of chiropractic was illegal! www.reggiegold.com

Sharon Gorman, D.C.

The enthusiasm Dr. Sharon Gorman has for Chiropractic is boundless. She actively practices its art, shares its philosophy, mentors its students, and serves on the board of Life University, where she graduated (1984). She does all these things in the service of advancing her profession, while also managing multiple high-volume practices where she shepherds young docs starting their careers. Dr. Gorman is co-founder of the League of Chiropractic Women (LCW), an organization dedicated to maximizing women's potential to balance the leadership of the profession she loves. Thanks to her tireless commitment, LCW provides leadership development for women in Chiropractic worldwide. www.gormanchiropractic.com www.lcwomen.com

Jessica Harden, D.C.

Dr. Jessica Harden is a solo female doc in Fort Mill, SC. Shortly after graduating she founded Providence Chiropractic and currently has one of the largest Pierce RESULTS System offices in the country. Dr. Jessica serves as a mentor on the AMPED team and travels to chiropractic campuses inspiring students and other doctors. She also has published studies on adolescent idiopathic scoliosis correction and is passionate about subluxation-based research. In 2016, she founded FLIGHT a program for women chiropractors designed to provide resources and build community support. When not in the office or traveling on the road, she spends time fishing with her husband, Stewart who is a professional kayak angler. www.providence-chiropractic.com www.flightconferences.com www.brandingyourcommunication.com/p/dr-jessica-harden

Amanda & Jeremy Hess, D.C.'s

Drs. Amanda & Jeremy Hess are devoted Chiropractors, Authors, and Serial Entrepreneurs whose Mission is to Help People Succeed by Living their Purpose and Finding Freedom. www.goDis coverHealth.com www.AmpedNow.com www.Rhinolife.org

Janice Hughes, D.C.

Dr. Janice Hughes has coached thousands of Chiropractors to success and profitability. After completing a successful biotech start up, Janice has turned her attention to creating Money Mindset online courses and '2Inspire Women' to increase the business savvy and entrepreneurial skills for all women in Chiropractic. www.drjanicehughes.com

D.D. Humber, D.C.

Dr. D.D. Humber is a 1956 graduate of Palmer College of Chiropractic. A long-time friend and associate of Dr. Sid Williams, D.D. has hosted the Dynamic Essentials Seminars since their inception over fifty years ago. Dr. Humber is a former Vice President of Life Chiropractic College, having joined the college in 1978. D.D. was named "Chiropractor of the Year" by the Georgia Chiropractic Association (1973) and by the Georgia Chiropractic Council (1998). Dr. Humber comes from a family comprised of many, many chiropractors dating back several decades.

Kevin Jackson and Selina Sigafoose-Jackson, D.C.'s

Drs. Kevin and Selina are both 1989 graduates of Life Chiropractic College in Marietta, GA. They've been in practice for thirty years and have two daughters Kinna and Kloe who are presently studying to be chiropractors themselves.
www.sigafoosejackson.com

Steve Judson, D.C.

Dr. Steve Judson has been practicing in Newington, Connecticut since 2002 and has a great passion for helping others reach their fullest potential through Chiropractic. He is a 1998 Life University graduate and has traveled around the world to Russia, Central America, Tobago, and the Dominican Republic educating doctors and patients about the power of the human body and its Innate wisdom to heal itself. As an upper cervical specialist, Dr. Judson trains chiropractors to become upper cervical specialists themselves. He speaks and educates internationally about people finding their destiny from within themselves. Dr. Judson prides himself most on his incredible family - his wife Tammy and his five beautiful children, Kylie, Sierra, Brooke, Kane, and Jaimee. Check out his new books **Atlas Adjusted** and **Wake Up Humans** at Amazon.com www.judsonchiropractic.com

Brian Kelly, D.C.

Dr. Brian Kelly is a chiropractor, speaker, and coach. He is a turnaround specialist having led transformational growth and change at two chiropractic colleges and a research organization. www.c1forsuccess.com

Christopher Kent, D.C.

Dr. Christopher Kent is a 1973 graduate of Palmer College of Chiropractic, and a diplomate and fellow of the ICA College of Chiropractic Imaging. He was named the International Chiropractors Association (ICA) "Chiropractic Researcher of the Year" in 1991 and ICA "Chiropractor of the Year" in 1998. Dr.

Kent is former chair of the United Nations NGO Health Committee, the first chiropractor elected to that office. Currently, Christopher is a professor and Director of Evidence-Informed Curriculum and Practice at Sherman College of Chiropractic. He does research on vertebral subluxation, wellness, and salutogenesis. A current project is "A Salutogenic Approach to Evidence-Informed Practice." www.sherman.edu

Daniel and Richelle Knowles, D.C.'s

Drs. Daniel and Richelle Knowles are known worldwide as a dynamic chiropractic husband-and-wife team. They are deeply committed to impacting the world for the better through chiropractic both by serving people in their office as well as helping chiropractic teams have more people — on more tables — more often.
www.networkwellnesscenters.com
www.lifetimewellnesspractice.com www.milehighchiro.org

Tedd Koren, D.C.

After graduating from Sherman College of Chiropractic (as class valedictorian) Dr. Tedd Koren jumped into private practice and professional involvement. He helped found Pennsylvania's only chiropractic college where he taught for nearly two years. Tedd is the most widely read Doctor of Chiropractic in the world today. Since 1987, when he started Koren Publications, over one hundred million pieces of his popular scientifically-referenced patient education materials have been distributed throughout the world. Dr. Koren founded the popular Koren Publications and the Koren Specific Technique. He lectures the world over and enjoys spending time with his wife Beth and their lovely family.
www.korenpublications.com www.korenwellness.com

Gilles LaMarche, D.C.

Dr. Gilles LaMarche is a chiropractor, educator, passionate healer, accomplished author, professional speaker, and inspiring certified personal development/executive coach. Gilles earned his Bachelor of Science from the University of Toronto and a Doctor

of Chiropractic degree from the Canadian Memorial Chiropractic College. Dr. LaMarche enjoyed private practice in Northern Ontario from 1979-2004, was named International Chiropractor of the Year by Parker Seminars in 1988, and Canadian Chiropractor of the Year for 2005-2006 by the readers of the Canadian Chiropractor magazine. From October 2006 to July 2012 he was a key member of the Parker University Executive team and in the fall of 2013 he joined the executive team at Life University as Vice President of Professional Relations.
www.life.edu www.facebook.com/gilles.lamarche

Larry Markson, D.C.

Dr. Larry Markson, started his career as a practicing chiropractor and ended up building one of the largest and most successful practices in the country. Over the next thirty-seven years he became a Personal Empowerment, Practice, Business Success and Prosperity Coach to over 30,000 people and has devoted his professional life to helping others transform their thoughts, actions, and feelings. He believes that your business and your personal life are waiting for a leader (YOU) to show up and that, "Who you are 'inside-the-skin' determines how well what you do works." Still going strong after five decades, he says his favorite creation is The Cabin Experience. He fully believes that success and happiness are "All In Your Head" and that "Success comes FROM you, not TO you." www.thecabinexperience.com

Ross McDonald and Rebecca Vickery, D.C.'s

Drs. Ross McDonald and his wife Dr. Rebecca Vickery are in private practice together in Edinburgh, Scotland. Together, they host The Edinburgh Lectures, an annual gathering of chiropractors and their teams in Edinburgh. He is the current President of the Scottish Chiropractic Association, Chair of the Board of Trustees tasked with developing a principled chiropractic degree program in Scotland, while Rebecca is an Executive Board member of the Scottish Chiropractic Association as it's treasurer.
www.chiropracticlectures.com www.scotlandcollegechiro.co.uk

The 8 Laws of Chiropractic Success

CJ Mertz, D.C.

By age twenty-eight, Dr. CJ Mertz had already built the largest healthcare practice in the world of its kind. Dr. Mertz gives all the credit to God for bringing to him the mentors he needed to help him reach his full potential. CJ founded Full Potential Leadership and XLR8 Coaching — the premiere business and chiropractic training organization. Since 1984, CJ has traveled more than three million miles, has taught more than 850 seminars, and has trained over sixteen thousand teams. www.cjmertz.com

Jeanne Ohm, D.C.

Dr. Jeanne Ohm has practiced family wellness care since 1981 with her husband, Dr. Tom. They have six children who were all born at home and are living the chiropractic family wellness lifestyle. Jeanne is Chief Executive Officer of the ICPA and Executive Editor of *Pathways to Family Wellness* magazine. An instructor, author, and innovator, her passion is training DC's on specific techniques for care in pregnancy, birth, and infancy. She focuses on forming national alliances for chiropractors with like-minded perinatal practitioners, empowering mothers to make informed choices, and offering pertinent patient educational materials. www.ohmchiropractic.com www.icpa4kids.com www.pathwaystofamilywellness.org

Paul Reed, D.C.

Dr. Paul Reed has been a practicing chiropractor for over twenty years. He had his first adjustment in the 8th grade and knew at that instant he wanted to be a chiropractor, even though he really had no idea what that meant. He followed this path through undergraduate school where he played Division 1, Pac 10 football. He began chiropractic school, literally 1 week following a bowl game his senior year. He opened his first practice in 1998. He has been blessed to be married twenty-five years, have two amazing children, run and operate four clinics, host one of the professions biggest gatherings, ChiroFEST and coach chiropractors to creating more in their lives! www.BridgeChirorpactic.com www.ChiroFEST.org www.DrPaulReed.com

Chuck Ribley, D.C.

Dr. Chuck "River" Ribley has spent a lifetime making a difference in chiropractic. He is a co-founder of Life University and was the spearhead in seeing it through its accreditation crisis in 2002. Dr. Ribley served for ten years on the Michigan Board of Chiropractic Examiners and founded the Michigan Association of Chiropractors where he led growth to over 2,000 members in just four years. Chuck also founded Inner Winners, a program designed to facilitate participants' ability to unleash their optimal potential by removing any interference they may be generating. In his "retirement," Dr. Ribley remains active and vital by serving as a consultant to the Life University Board of Trustees. He also adds to the growth of the profession through regular lectures to chiropractors and students in the USA, Europe, and Australia on the importance of chiropractic activism.
www.innerwinnersworldwide.com

Guy Riekeman, D.C.

Dr. Guy Riekeman obtained his chiropractic degree with honors in 1972 from Palmer College of Chiropractic in Iowa. He became a chiropractic spokesman, extolling the chiropractic message through award-winning television, video, and audio productions. As a leader for the chiropractic centennial celebration in 1995, he produced the nationally aired TV documentary "From Simple Beginnings," helping the public appreciate chiropractic's contribution to health and wellness. Guy was the fourth president of Life University in Marietta, Georgia and is currently Life University Chancellor. Dr. Riekeman continues to be highly sought as a motivational speaker at both the national and international levels.
ww.life.edu

Terry A. Rondberg, D.C.

After his graduation from Logan College of Chiropractic, Dr. Terry A. Rondberg built successful practices in St. Louis and Phoenix. He was noted for his emphasis on public and patient education and became a staunch advocate of subluxation-based chiropractic. As publisher of The Chiropractic Journal and founder and CEO of the World Chiropractic Alliance, he was a key figure in political lobbying, public education, and intra professional communication. He served on the Department of Defense Chiropractic Advisory Committee to help establish the protocol for making chiropractic services available to active duty military personnel. He also worked closely with global health care officials and organizations, including the World Health Organization.

Armand Rossi, D.C.

Dr. Armand Rossi is a 1976 graduate of Palmer College of Chiropractic. He has operated chiropractic clinics in Arizona, Florida, and Georgia. Armand is also a former instructor of Pediatric Adjusting at Life University in Marietta, GA. He is currently the Dean of Clinical Sciences at Sherman College of Chiropractic in Spartanburg, SC along with being a "Fellow" and teaching member of the International Chiropractic Pediatric Association, where he travels internationally bringing his chiropractic pediatric wisdom and expertise to chiropractors globally. He and his wife Terry live in South Carolina and have four children, eleven grandchildren, and eight great-grandchildren. www.sherman.edu

David K. Scheiner, D.C.

Originally from Queens, N.Y., Dr. David Scheiner is a 1996 graduate of Life Chiropractic College in Marietta, GA. He knew chiropractic was his calling when he sent away for information from Life College and while reading Dr. Sid Williams' presidents message in the college handbook in 1991, he had an awakening, where the universe called him to action to become a chiropractor. He fell in love with Dr. Sid's Native American and philosophical messages. He remained in Atlanta for twenty-two years after graduating in 1996 and opened four highly-successful chiropractic clinics with his wife Laura, a pediatric and pregnancy chiropractic specialist. In 2012, David went to work with Life Chiropractic College West in Hayward, CA and as Director of Recruitment helped take the college from 265 students to over 650 in under five years. He is a teacher of meditation, student of the esoteric and mystical arts, sought after lecturer, and author of two books — **Chiropractic Revealed**, an interview compilation including some of the most well-known chiropractors to ever grace the profession and — this volume, **The 8 Laws of Chiropractic Success.** David and his wife Laura currently reside in Phoenix, AZ and have three beautiful daughters; Megan, Kira, and Summer and two incredible dogs Charlie and Henri. www.davidscheiner.com

Frederick A. Schofield, D.C.

Dr. Frederick A. Schofield born in Cape Town, South Africa, has a uniqueness, excitement, and intensity about him, "One of a Kind." He is both player and coach, working in his office, and coaching chiropractors one on one. Teaching from 37+ years of proven fundamentals, Dr. Fred will open the door to a life of success, self-confidence, and boundless enthusiasm. Schofield Chiropractic Training Services mission is "To empower as many Chiropractors, as divinely possible, to improve their performance by expressing their potential; enhancing planet Earth and the health of humanity through applying and understanding the Principles of ChiropracTIC." www.MoChihChu.com

Liam Schubel, D.C.

Dr. Liam Schubel is a graduate of Life Chiropractic College and has been said to have "The Midas Touch" when it comes to Chiropractic Business. His business systems are being used by successful chiropractors worldwide to improve the efficiency, profitably, and impact of their chiropractic practices. He has also authored a critically acclaimed, international, smash hit book entitled CAST TO BE CHIROPRACTORS.
www.SchubelVisionElite.com
www.SchubelVisionWorldWide.com

James Sigafoose, D.C.

Dr. James Sigafoose is still known to many in the Chiropractic profession for his motivating and dynamic speeches and presentations. He was a devoted follower of the teachings of Dr.'s B.J. Palmer and Sid Williams, and his chiropractic philosophy and personal development seminars rang through the hallways of Chiropractors across the U.S. and internationally for five decades. A 1959 graduate of National Chiropractic College, he served on the boards of Life Chiropractic College and Life West. He lectured at numerous other chiropractic colleges, Parker Seminars, ICA conferences and Dynamic Essentials (DE). Dr. Sigafoose is also credited as offering the first Chiropractic Continuing Education Seminar. He is a legacy to Chiropractic professionally and personally. His passion filled his daily life, inspiring all six of his children, a son-in-law, a nephew, and a daughter-in-law to become chiropractors.
www.sigafoose.com

Joe Strauss, D.C.

A 1967 graduate of Columbia Institute of Chiropractic (now New York College of Chiropractic), Dr. Joe Strauss began private practice, and went on to also serve as a professor at Pennsylvania College of Chiropractic, teaching there from 1978 to 1994. He has served as Editor of *The Pivot Review*, a chiropractic philosophical publication, since 1983, and has written and published twenty books on the subject of chiropractic. In 1992 Dr. Strauss was elected a Fellow of the College of Straight Chiropractic, and in 1999 was honored as Chiropractor of the Year by Sherman College of Straight Chiropractic. He has lectured throughout the United States and overseas on the subject of straight chiropractic. He resides with his wife in Levittown, Pennsylvania, where he has maintained his large private practice for over 42 years.
www.chiropracticoutsidethebox.com

Teri and Stu Warner, D.C.'s

Drs. Teri & Stu Warner have revolutionized the chiropractic world by training and mentoring chiropractors to be the 'Go-To' kids health authority in their communities. Drs. Warner have been practicing for twenty-five years, are internationally sought after speakers, and regularly appear in the media, educating the world about raising healthy kids. Learn about the 12 building blocks to a world class pediatric practice at www.Chiropractic Pediatrics365.com

Tim Young, D.C.

Dr. Tim Young is the President of the Oklahoma Chiropractic Association and President of Focus OKC Chiropractic Educational seminars. Tim is also the President of Focus Foundations Chiropractic success coaching. He's married to his best friend Shannon who is his partner in everything. Tim is the father of three and grandfather to one, while still maintaining one of the most successful Chiropractic practices in the world. www.Focusokc.com

Conclusion

Chiropractic was founded on a principle of tone. There is a vibration streaming throughout the entire universe, which courses through each animated and inanimate object. At present, this vibration of love is mostly stuck, as the consciousness of humanity is wrapped around the theme of pain and suffering. We see evidence of this in the wildfires, mass shootings, massive floods, opioid epidemic, and myriad of other global upheaval.

Chiropractic was founded by D.D. Palmer, D.C., a spiritualist who was given this gift and had the intention that every man, woman, and child receive the wondrous benefits of the chiropractic adjustment in order to be in-tune with and the fullest expression of themselves.

Observing the current global affairs and individual internal affairs, it's safe to say that what D.D. had in mind is not what is occurring today. You became (or are becoming) a chiropractor to break out of the mold of what's normal and ordinary, not to attempt to find ways to fit into that model. You must be bold, daring, and willing to shift your mindset into something completely new in order to experience the extraordinary.

The same way birds know how to fly north in the summer and south in the winter, you have within you an internal compass that is always pointing to your purpose, passion, and direction in life. The time has come for you to connect to your internal GPS and get on the path of joy, happiness, and success in both your chiropractic and personal Life. Perhaps you thought chiropractic was the right profession and have come to question whether that is true. Be real with yourself so you may in turn be true to others. If you're struggling, it's ok to get vulnerable and ask one of the leaders in this book for help. Our website information is listed in the contributor bio section. We'd Love to help you — for loving's sake.

A good friend of mine and I grew up together in Roslyn, Long Island. His name is Jesse Itzler and he's the Author of the best-selling book **Living With A Seal**. He says, "How you do anything is how you do everything." I want you to start taking inventory of your life and your practice today. Take each item you write down and ask the question, "Do I Love spending my time doing this?" and "Do I Love spending the time with the people I'm spending my time with?" The answers to those two questions will reveal a lot for you and determine much of your future happiness.

This book's sole aim is for you to come away with the ability to live a life you love and live it powerfully on your terms. What will you create for yourself now? What results are you setting out to accomplish? You must create what's next with your life and be willing to jump forward into the abyss of what's NEW. Look through the front windshield instead of the rear.

What's available for you if you choose to practice and live your life in alignment with your wildest dreams? Allow yourself to be touched, moved, and inspired each time you pull up to your chiropractic practice and your home, for you know that it is you who is going to be of service to both your practice members and your family. How are you going to show up?

Take some time for yourself each day (personal time) to reflect on your business and personal life. Take account for all the buckets of your life and observe the ways of behaving and acting that may be inauthentic. Be completely authentic about where you've been being inauthentic in your Life and begin to take action in order to have transformation in your chiropractic practice and Life.

More knowledge isn't the missing piece for you. The answers you seek are found within **The 8 Laws of Chiropractic Success** and in the day to day moments as your life is unfolding. This is where you'll find your peace, bliss, and eternal success.

Go and share with others what you're out to newly achieve

and discover. It may be unknown for you so I invite you to reflect on and discover internal sources and resources of your beauty and the truth of your being.

Yes, imagination has mostly become abandoned in our world today. Yet, it is this Living Imagination where self-innovation and self-transformation will arise for you and it's also the platform where creative self-discovery and inventions emerge. What will you discover? What will you invent?

My friends, this isn't a practice life. It's the only one you have. So, take out a mirror, hold it up, and discover the beautiful soul that is you. Now go out and share it with the world!

Made in the USA
Columbia, SC
08 June 2018